Toward a Bet

Advance Praise for *Toward a Better World*

Dr. Mark Lazenby presents a profound moral and practical philosophy, exemplified in the everyday caring practices of nurses *doing for* and *being with* others in response to our shared humanity, vulnerability, and a quest for thriving. He argues that our moral obligations to the earth and to one another precede rights and, when fulfilled, create a better, richer, and more sustainable human existence for all. This book is a testament to belonging to our fellow human beings and Earth.

Patricia Benner, PhD, RN, FAAN
Professor Emeritus
School of Nursing
University of California, San Francisco

In *Toward a Better World*, Mark Lazenby makes a compelling case to view nursing as a moral profession with an inherent social contract to contribute to humanity. By expanding the scope of the intimate nature of healing that is central to the practice of nursing, we are asked to step up and contribute to dignity on both a local and global scale. Given there are twenty million nurses worldwide, with this potential, how can we not? There is pain in these words but also hope, and these are words we need to hear. So while Lazenby honors nursing and its many contributions, he calls us to courage—and to be more. This is a book that needs to be read by the profession, by those who seek to join its ranks, and by leaders in all the health professions who have the potential to unite and enact a social and moral response to the current health inequities that puzzle and besiege us.

Professor Suzanne Chambers, AO
Dean and Professor
Faculty of Health
University of Technology Sydney

In *Toward a Better World*, Mark Lazenby has extended Lilian Wald's early twentieth-century vision—of working with the community, of understanding the problems of the poor, and of being committed to social and economic equality—to eloquently and convincingly make the case for nursing's mission in working toward a better world. He has taken us further, still, to the words and actions of modern nursing's first ethicist, Annie Goodrich, who also reminded us not to forget our obligations "to change the conditions of ill-health and bad-living." Goodrich envisioned "the City Beautiful." In this volume, Lazenby leads us to a better and more beautiful world.

Deborah Chyun, PhD, RN, FAAN, FAHA
Dean and Professor
University of Connecticut School of Nursing

In this important discourse of philosophy in nursing, Dr. Lazenby challenges us as nurses to work together for a better world and shapes for us a vision for modern nursing. Since the origins of our profession, nurses have not shied away from issues of social, political, and economic inequality but engaged with a powerful voice for social justice. Fortunately, as a profession we have discarded a history of patriarchy and the fetters of social hierarchy to have a powerful voice at decision-making tables. Dr. Lazenby's book is appropriate and timely as nurses emerge from stereotypical roles in hospitals to take places of leadership. No matter where nurses work, a defining feature of the practice of all nurses is a responsibility to care for others and a commitment to ensuring health for all —this moving text provides an inspirational blueprint.

Patricia M. Davidson, PhD, RN, FAAN
Dean and Professor
Johns Hopkins University School of Nursing

Toward a Better World, by Dr. Mark Lazenby, reminds each of us why we entered this sacred profession of nursing. It should be read by every practicing nurse and should be required reading for every nursing student. The stories in this book, told through the eyes that only a nurse could have, remind us of the common good and all the forces in the world that now threaten that good. Every page of the book is profound, but my favorite words are in the preface as Dr. Lazenby writes, "I feel helpless but I am not helpless. I am a nurse."

Betty Rollins Ferrell, PhD, CHPN, FAAN, FPCN
Director and Professor
Division of Nursing Research and Education
City of Hope

"[T]o make the world a better place." This is the challenge and the imperative that Dr. Mark Lazenby lays out for the reader and for the nursing profession in his second book on the ethical and social significance of nursing. At a time when nationalism, climate damage, and other planetary stressors threaten the best of *Homo sapiens'* achievements, he reminds us of the human connection that is crucial and that is intrinsic to nursing as a discipline and practice. In doing so, he urges those of us who are nurses to our better selves, and indeed makes the case that this aspiration is fundamental for all humans to appreciate if we are to save our families, communities, and the world itself in the coming decades. His clarion call is timely and tender. We ignore it at our peril. Read this book and be (re)inspired about what is possible through nursing, and through nursing our societies back to health.

Ann Kurth, PhD, RN, MPH, FAAN
Dean and Linda Koch Professor
Yale University School of Nursing

Nurse-philosopher Lazenby's *Toward a Better World* is a companion piece to his ethics book *Caring Matters Most*. Confronting the turmoil of current times, he argues for the importance of nursing as a force for global societal change because of the profession's fundamental obligations—to promote equality, peace, and respect; provide assistance and safety; and protect the earth's integrity. By seizing on large global themes, he arms nurses with principled reasons to lead, but he also makes clear that these righteous stances are always played out locally. When ethical principles energize the particular, the social significance of nursing is clear—and this can provide the needed force for change.

Angela Barron McBride, PhD, RN, FAAN
Distinguished Professor and University Dean Emerita
Indiana University School of Nursing

Dr. Lazenby weaves personal stories with references of history, philosophy, and sociology to create a call to action for nurses in *Toward a Better World: The Social Significance of Nursing*. The book is organized in sections, first a discussion of nursing as moral profession and then deeper exploration of nursing's obligations of equality, assistance, peace, safety, care of Earth, and respect. He writes with optimism as a nurse and knowledge that nursing, the largest profession in the world, has the power to create a good society and make the world a better place. This is a book that not only is a gift to read and think deeply about the messages but also is perfect for discussion in the classroom or book club.

Brenda Nevidjon
Chief Executive Officer
Oncology Nursing Society

Dr. Lazenby's book is simultaneously a tribute to nursing as a moral endeavor, evoking pride in the profession, and a call to action. It serves as a declaration of why the voice of nursing needs to be included in public discourse at all levels and on all relevant issues, while also calling out the obligation of every nurse to advocate publicly on every measure that affects human well-being. He makes the case with conceptual rigor and through compelling narrative. While recalling acts of great courage by specific nurses, he also honors everyday practice, demonstrating how the act of nursing itself, in all its forms, is a powerful force for good in the world. It is a book all nurses should read and a message the world needs to hear.

Douglas P. Olsen, PhD, RN
Associate Professor, Michigan State University College of Nursing & College of Human Medicine
Associate Professor, Sechenov University, Moscow, Russian Federation
Contributing Editor, *American Journal of Nursing*

In *Toward a Better World: The Social Significance of Nursing*, Dr. Lazenby makes a compelling case for the essential role nursing should play in addressing key social issues. As health care delivery becomes increasingly complex and technological, this important text re-establishes our professional responsibility to treat others with compassion, dignity, and respect and situates the duty to care as a moral imperative for nurses worldwide.

Richard Ricciardi, PhD, CRNP, FAAN
Professor, George Washington University
President, Sigma Theta Tau International
Professor, The George Washington University School of Nursing

In this inspiring work, Lazenby reveals the soul of the nurse and exposes us all to the potential of the nursing collective to address the universal good. With personal stories of nurses and a remarkable historical perspective, he reminds us of our core contract with society not only to do good locally but also to reinforce our collective force to commit to issues of our times that threaten the well-being and health of the human condition. Through caring for the earth, engaging with peace, living with respect, and radical equity, Lazenby lights a re-envisioned humanistic value for all nurses and society to embrace!

Eileen Sullivan-Marx
President, American Academy of Nursing
Dean and Erline Perkins McGriff Professor
Rory Myers College of Nursing
New York University

Benjamin Franklin proposed that "the noblest question in the world is . . . What good may I do in it?" Mark Lazenby addresses a similarly important question for the nursing profession—its role in bringing about a good society. Drawing on philosophy, history, and his personal and professional reflections, Lazenby not only raises more questions but also provides direction to how we might think about our obligations to humanity. This book is an important frame as the profession of nursing raises its voice in addressing health equity, social determinants of health, climate change, and other challenges in the twenty-first century.

Antonia M. Villarruel, PhD, RN, FAAN
Professor and Margaret Bond Simon Dean of Nursing
Senior Fellow, Leonard Davis Institute of Health Economics
University of Pennsylvania School of Nursing

Toward a Better World is truly captivating, leaving the reader savoring the kernel and deliberateness of every sentence. It is powerfully validating and thought provoking, inspiring all of us to actively engage in advancing the social significance of nursing for the greater good of the world.

Barbara E. Wolfe, PhD, RN, FAAN
Dean and Professor
College of Nursing
The University of Rhode Island

Toward a
Better World

The Social Significance of Nursing

MARK LAZENBY, PHD, APRN, FAAN

University of Connecticut School of Nursing

Oxford University Press

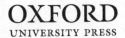

OXFORD
UNIVERSITY PRESS

OXFORD
UNIVERSITY PRESS

Oxford University Press is a department of the University of Oxford. It furthers
the University's objective of excellence in research, scholarship, and education
by publishing worldwide. Oxford is a registered trade mark of Oxford University
Press in the UK and certain other countries.

Published in the United States of America by Oxford University Press
198 Madison Avenue, New York, NY 10016, United States of America.

© Oxford University Press 2020

CIP data is on file at the Library of Congress
ISBN 978-0-19-069571-2

This material is not intended to be, and should not be considered, a substitute for medical or
other professional advice. Treatment for the conditions described in this material is highly
dependent on the individual circumstances. And, while this material is designed to offer
accurate information with respect to the subject matter covered and to be current as of the
time it was written, research and knowledge about medical and health issues is constantly
evolving and dose schedules for medications are being revised continually, with new side
effects recognized and accounted for regularly. Readers must therefore always check the
product information and clinical procedures with the most up-to-date published product
information and data sheets provided by the manufacturers and the most recent codes of
conduct and safety regulation. The publisher and the authors make no representations or
warranties to readers, express or implied, as to the accuracy or completeness of this material.
Without limiting the foregoing, the publisher and the authors make no representations or
warranties as to the accuracy or efficacy of the drug dosages mentioned in the material. The
authors and the publisher do not accept, and expressly disclaim, any responsibility for any
liability, loss or risk that may be claimed or incurred as a consequence of the use and/or
application of any of the contents of this material.

3 5 7 9 8 6 4 2

Printed by Marquis, Canada

Disclaimer

The stories I have told in this book are based on my experiences. I have changed the identities of some people when I have not been able to obtain their permission to use their real names, mostly because of their deaths or when I have had no way to contact them. However, I tell the stories as truthfully as my memory allows.

*For Carl—a nurse who has made the world
a better place on two continents*

Contents

Foreword

In May 2019, the World Health Assembly will declare 2020 as the "Year of the Nurse and the Midwife," also marking the two hundredth anniversary of the birth of Florence Nightingale, the founder of modern nursing. This declaration will be one of those once-in-a-generation opportunities to put nurses and midwives at the center of global and national health policies, and to celebrate what nurses and midwives do to improve health and health care in their communities and across the world. It comes with the realization and conviction that developing nursing and midwifery, and allowing nurses and midwives to work to their full potential, is one of the most important things we can do to improve health globally and achieve universal health coverage.

The author of this book on the social significance of nursing espouses these very values of developing nursing and midwifery to achieve universal health coverage. For millions of people across the world, the only health worker they will ever be seen, counseled, and treated by is a nurse or midwife. This role of caring for all people, regardless of who they are, by reaching some of the most marginalized communities is essential to leaving no one behind and achieving health for all. This is what the author describes as caring and working for the common good.

In describing this common good, the author gives an example of a good society as shown by two nurses in a very short-staffed clinic in Botswana but who operate under the spirit of *Botho*: a philosophy and way of life whereby all are respected, differences are tolerated, and everyone generally enjoys good positive regard from others in the family, the community, the village, and beyond. Being from Botswana, I can relate to that; and it is this spirit of *Botho* that forms the basis of Mark Lazenby's six obligations that the nursing profession has to the human community: equality, assistance, peace, safety, care for Earth, and respect for ourselves and others.

I am honored to write this foreword for a book whose story I have lived and witnessed as a nurse. As the cochair of the Nursing Now global campaign, I espouse the very values of caring and working for the common good. Nursing Now is a global campaign that aims to improve health and health care globally by raising the status and profile of nurses and midwives. The campaign is working with partners to champion influential leadership roles for nurses and midwives. Being influential leaders means that they will be able to apply their own experiences as well as evidence and data to stimulate changes in policy and improve health care delivery. We work to empower nurses to take their place at the heart of tackling twenty-first-century health challenges. By influencing policy at global and national levels, we aim to increase investment in nursing and midwifery, improve global and national policies on nursing and midwifery, strengthen nurse leadership and influence at all levels, and encourage the sharing of effective practice across the world.

This book speaks the language of Nursing Now and contributes to the dialogue around health care practices in a fast-globalizing world where nurse leaders have to manage issues of gender equality, sexual orientation, and cultural and other diversity. Very few books exist for mentoring young people upon entering the caring professions, so this book will assist in filling that void. The anecdotes, the lessons learned, and the questions at the end are valuable and need to be shared with many others who may not have male and female role models and mentors to initiate them into the tough reality of the caring world.

This book is a must read because it is an experiential, nonfiction narrative that will definitely change the practice and perspectives of nurses and midwives. In describing the six obligations that the nursing profession has to the human community, Mark Lazenby gives a basis and motivational grounding for some of the best practices in workplace human resource policies for sustainable development, of how best to recruit, nurture, retain, and manage nursing talent in today's fast-growing and globalized economy. Narrated examples would include targeted staff development, ethical decision making, policies for the prevention of harassment, easing the burden of unpaid care work, and mentoring junior nurses through targeted development.

In June 2019, at the International Council of Nurses (ICN) Congress in Singapore, the ICN will launch the Nightingale Challenge. This initiative calls for all employers of nurses and midwives globally to provide development opportunities in influential leadership for young nurses and midwives during 2020, to build their skills as advocates and influential leaders in health care. Unless nursing is rapidly expanded and developed, it will be impossible to achieve the World Health Assembly goal of a billion more people benefiting from universal health coverage within five years. The world needs thinkers like Mark Lazenby to inspire and motivate the young nurses to become those very advocates and influential leaders of Agenda 2030, the United Nations' plan "to ensure that all human beings can fulfill their potential in dignity and equality and in a healthy environment."

Professor Sheila Dinotshe Tlou
Cochair, Nursing Now; Professor Emerita,
University of Botswana; Member, US National Academy
of Medicine; Former Director of UNAIDS for Eastern and
Southern Africa; Former Minister of Health of Botswana
April 2019

Preface

Recently, the government of the United States, my country, shut down for the longest period ever. The morning newspaper told of federal workers, deprived of their pay, standing in line for free meals. The chef who provided these meals usually does so only during natural disasters; that government workers found themselves without money to buy food *was* a disaster, he said. The shutdown was due to disagreement over building a wall along the US border to keep people out: xenophobia had brought the world's foremost democracy to a standstill.

At the same time, the difficulty of extracting the United Kingdom from the European Union paralyzed the UK government. The United Kingdom was going to "take back control" of its borders, said the campaign to leave the European Union. Meanwhile, all across Europe, overt violent expressions of prejudice are on the rise, giving nationalist and racist movements publicity that would have been unthinkable only a few years ago.

While this discord continues in the comfortable West, war rages in Syria, whose citizens—maimed, starving, displaced, and traumatized—just want the conflict to end. Around the world, extremists kill soldiers and citizens alike in bomb attacks. In Myanmar, a country headed by a Nobel Peace Prize laureate, the Rohingya people flee their homeland in the face of massacre by government forces. Meanwhile, in the United States, the richest couple ever have announced they are divorcing. Speculation about how they will divide their $150 billion fortune fascinates in a way that the thirteen million hungry children living in the United States simply do not. And all the while, Earth's climate is changing disastrously because of our use of fossil fuels. If I dwell on these, and other, dissonances of this time, I feel helpless.

But I am not helpless. I am a nurse, and nurses are anything but helpless.

We nurses are not helpless when we encounter a patient in crisis. We are not helpless when a baby decides to be born. Nor are we helpless when another nurse needs a hand. If we happen upon an accident, we fulfill our duty of care, and even if there may not be anything we can do, we are present. Just as we are not helpless in our usual duties, I do not think that we should feel helpless against the dissonances of this, or any, time. Rather, I think that as nurses we have a duty to respond to the social ills of our time.

Our response is to care about these ills. Caring is at the heart of the nursing profession. We care for the sick and vulnerable in the most intimate of ways. This is nursing's creed: to care for the other when the other cannot care for him- or herself. This caring makes nursing a moral profession. People see this morality and respond to it by saying, year after year, that nurses are the most trusted of all professions. As the profession with the most members world-wide, nursing can use its morality, and the trust people put in nurses, to respond to social ills—indeed, as it has in every genera-tion. However, in this book I make the case that nursing's morality requires more than responding to social ills.

It requires that nursing works for the common good. We can work for a better world for ourselves, our families, our communities, and our countries, but as nurses, whose mandate is to care for all people regardless of who they are, we ought to consider ourselves as citizens of the world: our work is for all. As nurses, we do not merely care for individuals here and there; rather, the collection of nurses that is the profession of nursing worldwide cares for the entire human community. This is this book's central argument: by working for the common good, through fulfilling our obligations to the entire human community, and that which sustains the human community, the profession of nursing works toward a better world—for all.

In what follows, I describe six obligations the profession has to the human community: equality, assistance, peace, safety, care for Earth, and respect for ourselves and others. My description of these obligations is nothing new. In fact, it is common sense. But what is new is the view that, by fulfilling them, the profession of nursing can use its power—the power of being the most trusted and the largest profession—to work toward a better world, even amid the social ills of this or any time. Nursing is more than caring for individuals; its work is for the common good—the good society for all.

Nursing has been a harbinger of the good society throughout its modern history. The profession of nursing has given women— when disenfranchised and with few options for education and work—a legitimate career by which to rise out of poverty and make a livable wage, to gain an education, and to have a profession. By doing all this, long before suffrage in most Western countries, nursing opened possibilities for women. Mary Wollstonecraft, with her 1792 *A Vindication of the Rights of Women,* ushered in what is called the first wave of feminism. Between Wollstonecraft and what is known as the second wave of feminism, which began in the mid-twentieth century, stood Florence Nightingale. If not in full agreement with feminists of her era, Nightingale argued for women's emancipation from the strictures of a sexist society, and she argued that the profession of nursing was one way to do that. Indeed, nursing, I believe, has made it possible for women to be considered capable of being scientists—nurse scientists or otherwise—of being doctors, lawyers, engineers, and high-ranking academics of all sorts. For instance, the first woman president of an Ivy League university in the United States was a nurse, Claire Fagin, who served as president of the University of Pennsylvania. Nursing has been doing for women while doing for others. Do for others, and you shall do for yourself. That is what Annie Goodrich did by opening, in 1923, the first university-based nursing school in the world, the Yale School of Nursing. As the first woman to be a dean at Yale, she paved the way for women to be admitted to the university's under-graduate programs, which were men-only until 1968. Her modus operandi was to do for women while doing for the profession. Just as nursing has done for women, so too nursing can do for society.

Nursing focuses on the other—the other who is a patient, the other that is a family, a neighborhood, a community, a country, and in so doing, the entire human community. Nursing, with its outward focus, eschews the inward focus of the present times—the times of "Take *my* country back," of nationalism and racism, of widening income inequality, of a degrading climate. An inward-focused approach to society will not—cannot—result in a better society; it can only result in exclusion and xenophobia, in greed, in continuing climate change, all of which militate against working to-ward a better world. A world better than the world of the present is one in which people care for the well-being of their fellow human and one that sustains all humans. To work toward a better world, one must be other focused, as nursing has always been.

When I see what nursing has achieved in the past, I think that the profession has a chance to work for a better world in the pre-sent. After all, a better world is not realized in some mythical future when all things are made right. A better world comes about in the struggle—in incremental progress. Nursing, in the 150-plus years of its modern history, has been part of that progress. Evidence of past progress, made through nurses caring about the human com-munity, gives us hope to continue to work toward a better world in the present.

Nurses are not helpless. Rather, we see what needs to be done, and we do it. My *cri de couer* in this book is for the profession to see what needs to be done with the big social issues of our time (and in future times) and, with the power of the trust the human community places in the profession and on the grand scale that the profession's size permits, to do what needs to be done. After all, there is no utopia that will one day materialize if we only work hard enough. Rather, it is the act of working for the good of all, right now, that in itself makes the world a better place—now and in the future.

Acknowledgments

The size of this small book, as with its predecessor, *Caring Matters Most*, is inversely proportioned to the care and thought placed in every argument, every sentence, every word. The writing has come slowly and deliberately. Dear reader, please read it with the same slowness and deliberateness. For your care in reading, I acknowledge you. I also acknowledge that you may not agree with every thought or sentence, every argument or sentiment. But I hope that in your disagreement you too will acknowledge that it has stimulated your own thoughts and arguments about how the profession of nursing—indeed, how any helping profession—has the power to make the world a better place.

My own thoughts have been stimulated by my exceedingly bright students at Yale School of Nursing (YSN), where I worked when I wrote this book. Stephen Breazeale, Michael Anthony Moore, Patrick Richardson, Abigail Wilpers, the Doctor of Nursing Practice students in my ethics courses in 2017, 2018, and 2019— you have all sharpened my thoughts and arguments, and hence, made this a better book. To YSN dean and professor emeritus Judith Krauss, the Helen Porter Jayne and Martha Prosser Jayne professor emeritus Marjorie Funk (their emeritus status indicates their wisdom and thus the degree to which they have made this a better book), and lecturer Judith Kunisch: for reading the manuscript in stages and pointing me to a straighter path, thank you. To my dean at YSN when I wrote the book, Ann Kurth, for reading parts and for her support, I am grateful. I am especially indebted to my then-chairperson, Professor M. Tish Knobf, who has read the manuscript several times, given constructive feedback, and provided encouragement along the way. Tish, when I had doubts about this book project, after talking with you, I had faith; I am so very appreciative.

Ruth McCorkle, the Florence Schorske Wald professor emeritus at Yale, has been my mentor for over a decade. She is the one who, not just through her research but also through her teaching and her nursing practice, has shown me the truth of what I write. For this, my indebtedness to her cannot be repaid.

To the Faculty of Health, particularly the nurses, at the University of Technology Sydney, who listened to the chapter on safety and gave me feedback; the cancer rehabilitation nurses in Mumbai, Varanasi, and Delhi, India; the nurses at the King Hussein Cancer Center in Amman, Jordan, especially Ghadeer Alarja; and the nurses in Gaborone, Botswana, especially to Dr. Norman Carl Swart, to whom this book is dedicated—thank you. You all have taught me how my nursing practice makes the world a better place. You are the good society.

I am especially grateful to Professor Sheila Tlou, who has dedicated her nursing practice to bettering the world, for taking the time and care to write a foreword.

To my editors at Oxford University Press: First, I owe much to Rebecca Suzan, who took the proposal under her care and shepherded it through the process. This is our third book together, and now that she has moved on, I feel her loss. Second, to Lucy Randall and her assistant, Hannah Doyle, who deftly picked up the shepherding of the manuscript through final reviews, production, and onward, I give my gratitude.

Leonie Gombrich—who was the governor of a primary school during the editing of this book, continues to be the literary executor of the twentieth century's most celebrated and important art historian, and is a mother and wife, in the course of her doing all this good—has taken interest in my arguments and the prose in which I try to convey them. There is no greater partnership in the scholarly enterprise than that between a writer and an editor. Thank you, Leonie; you are not only a world-class editor but also a scholar.

These wonderful people have helped me, but all errors and lapses are mine alone—that is for sure.

I owe a special debt of gratitude to my current dean, Deborah A. Chyun, for her mentorship, first when I was becoming a nurse, and now under her leadership.

In nursing, books are written at the expense of family, for they are written after all the science tasks are done. To my wife, Jodi, and my son, Ethan, and to the newest member of our family who tells me, by placing his paw on my arm, when the night is late and it is bedtime: I hope that the time I have spent away from you writing this book will, in the end, be worth it, for, after all, I hope that what I have done here will make the world that much better for you and for us together. At the end of the day, loved ones matter most. Thank you, Jodi and Ethan, for your patience and support. I give you all my love and the fruits of my endeavors.

Finally, it bears mentioning that the late Donna Diers, a former dean and professor at YSN, suggested to me in 2008, when I was still training to be a nurse, that I should bring Annie Goodrich's volume on the ethical and social significance of nursing into the twenty-first century. Donna, I have tried to do this with *Caring Matters Most: The Ethical Significance of Nursing* and *Toward a Better World: The Social Significance of Nursing*.

It is now up to you to judge if I have succeeded.

1

Nursing and the Good Society

It was the summer of 2007. I was in southern Africa to study death and the human immunodeficiency virus (HIV). I had traveled a day's drive outside the city where I was working to a rural health post that served a village of fewer than a thousand people. At that health post, I encountered two nurses. They were young men, probably in their midtwenties. One sported dreadlocks down to his midback. Both wore stud earrings. Except for their all-white nursing uniforms, they could have been two young men in Los Angeles, London, or New York. But instead, they were in that rural village staffing the two-room health post. They lived in a small house behind it. And they did everything. They conducted physical exams and took blood and other specimens and shipped them off to the faraway lab. They prescribed and dispensed medications. Much to my surprise, they were also midwives; they brought babies into the world and then provided their well-baby care. They were the one-stop shop for health care in that village. And it was unrelenting work: they were on duty twenty-four/seven. I marveled at their skill, knowledge, and fortitude. I called them "supernurses." But I wondered how they could devote themselves to such demanding and nonstop care of the people of that village, especially when, at their age, one would expect them to be in the city having a good time after work. After all, when I was in the city, the malls, restaurants, and pubs were full of young adults who looked just like them enjoying themselves in their free time. But these two young men did not have the time or luxury to go out after work. They had dedicated their lives to nursing in a way I had not previously understood.

In a lull—I had sat there for hours enthralled, watching them see one patient after another—I asked them how they could do all this. Almost in unison, they answered, "Because we owe it to our people." They then went on to tell me how they had grown up during the time when there were no antiretroviral medications to treat HIV; these medications had become widely available only a few years earlier. They had watched their loved ones—including one of their own mothers—die of HIV-related diseases. They did what they were doing because they thought their work could further what the antiretroviral medications had done: contribute to a better society.

What is the nursing profession's role in bringing about a good society? What, if anything, does the profession of nursing owe to society? These two questions are the subject of this book.

The good society, the twentieth-century sociologist Robert Bellah said, rests in the institutions necessary for people to live good lives. For people to be able to live good lives, these institutions must also be good. Bellah's contemporary, the philosopher John Rawls, thought much the same: a good society is structured around good political and social institutions. Good political institutions ensure the equality of basic liberties, and good social institutions ensure the equality of opportunity. Citizens of a good society, Rawls said, must accept the principles by which these good political and social institutions operate. For both Bellah and Rawls, good institutions structure the good society.

The good society, according to one of the twentieth century's most influential economists, John Kenneth Galbraith, affords all its members access to a rewarding life through economic means: financial security for older adults, unemployment compensation for the jobless, a livable minimum wage, and more taxes on the rich than the poor are among the economic measures that Galbraith proposed as necessary to enable access to a rewarding life. Galbraith also foretold the time we find ourselves in today, a time in which the nation-state is too narrow a view for these economic measures.

More than ever, we live in a multilateral world. The production of goods and the offering of services no longer rest in one nation. An automobile, for example, is made of parts produced in several countries, and the final product is assembled in yet other countries. When I call for assistance with my computer or my phone, I will more than likely speak to someone who is separated from me by an ocean. People in these other countries, just as people in my country, deserve access to the economic means necessary for a rewarding life. After all, that which makes a society good is common to all humans regardless of their nationality. This makes sense. What is good for one here is good for another there. Adam Smith, the eighteenth-century Scottish philosopher who founded the discipline of economics, suggested this more than three hundred years ago. What is good for the individual is good for everyone.

The freedom for the individual to be and to do that of which he or she is capable is necessary for the good society, according to the Nobel economist and philosopher Amartya Sen. Of course, this freedom is for all individuals, regardless of where they live.

When one becomes a nurse, one cannot help but ask the question of what is a good society. Nurses see the effects of the ills of society more often than they see the good. In urgent care and emergency departments, in diabetes and cancer clinics, in primary care offices and schools, and in psychiatric offices and hospitals, nurses see the effects of disease and misfortune. They also see the effects of war and violence and of homelessness, hunger, and food insecurity, among other physically and emotionally debilitating effects of poverty, discrimination, and lack of education. Once these effects are seen, it is impossible to ignore the question of what is necessary for a society not to have these ills. I often hear nurses ask the question of what needs to be done to address the root causes of why their patients are in the emergency department, the hospital, or the clinic. "If only there were somewhere the homeless could be fed and sheltered, they wouldn't need to come to the hospital." "If inner-city dwellers had somewhere to buy fresh fruit and vegetables, would we see this much obesity?" In these "ifs" lies the fundamental question: What is necessary for a good society?

This has long been a question—and a motivating one—for nurses. The founder of the modern profession of nursing, Florence Nightingale, pressed for reforms in British workhouses. In nineteenth-century England, workhouses were places where people who were unable to support themselves were offered room and board in return for work. In practice, they were often little better than labor camps. The poor in these institutions, Nightingale said, needed proper nursing and infirmaries when they were sick. These improvements, she proposed to members of the British Parliament and influential people in her country, should be paid for by a tax. Of equal importance to her was decreasing the numbers of the poor who were imprisoned in workhouses. In letters to the high and mighty, even the monarch, she implored people to address sources of poverty. And along with this, she took up the cause of ending child labor. The good society, to Nightingale, was one in which nurses cared for the poor and the vulnerable while working to eradicate the causes of their poverty and vulnerability. Nightingale, in her time and within her context, asked the question of what nursing ought to do to foster the good society.

I ask Nightingale's question within the time I am writing. It is a time of war and the devastation of war; and yet, it is a time when more people than ever live in peace. It is a time of violence, which in my own country is often rooted in a long history of racial injustice; yet it is a time when people of color are the majority population worldwide, and for the first time in the 240-plus years of my country's history, a person of color was elected to the presidency— twice. It is a time of great income inequality, but fewer people live in extreme poverty. It is a time of refugees and migrants fleeing war and economic insecurity; but it is also a time when, in the richest countries of the world, we have the means to harbor migrants fleeing economic insecurity and war. It is also a time when the climate is rapidly changing due to human behavior, altering the environment necessary for life; and yet science and technology offer innovations that, along with more ecologically sustainable lifestyles, can slow if not reverse this change.

It is a time during which we possess the knowledge to address the ills of society—a time during which we know what must be done and how to do it to bring about a good society. But it is also a time when progress threatens established self-interests. As some organizations work for social and economic conditions that address global poverty, others, including nation-states, retreat into isolation. As they do, economic classes become insulated from each other, and the rich grow unfathomably richer. Clean, renewable, and more efficient energy technologies offer a framework for a livable climate. Communities and individuals around the world have adopted these technologies as well as lifestyles that stay within the limits of our natural world. And yet powerful lobbies seek to protect the profitability of industries that militate against the collective promise of these new technologies and sustainable lifestyles. These (and other) examples suggest the age during which I write this book: an age when we care about societal ills and have solutions to address them but the powers of self-interest frustrate our care.

These opposing forces of caring and self-interest notwithstanding, I believe that our natural inclination is to care for each other. The contemporary social psychologist Dacher Keltner has argued convincingly that humanity would not have survived its long evolutionary journey without concern for the other. I also believe that, today, the prevailing attitude is to care for the human community and the planet that sustains life. But equally, self-interest—toward national identities, toward amassing wealth, toward personal comfort and ease, and toward the individual—threatens progress toward a good society; that is, care-lessness about societal problems often trumps care. The polarities of care versus care-lessness typify the time in which I write.

Nursing gives a forum in which this polarity *can* dissolve. In nursing, knowledge about how to improve society meets application of that knowledge. It is in this way that the care of nursing is moral: it brings an orientation toward the whole over the care-lessness of self-interest. Through acts of caring, nursing brings what is right to that which needs to be righted. Nursing brings good into society.

Some may protest that the profession's primary responsibility is not to care for the big problems of our time but rather to care for individuals, families, and populations. It is true that nurses care for individuals, families, and populations, and it has long been recognized that to do this, nurses must be concerned with the conditions of daily life that affect health. However, this is not a book about the social determinants of health. Economic, social, political, and environmental conditions necessary for health are not the sum of what is necessary for a good society. Following Sen, the good society is that which is necessary for people to live a good life, a life in which they are free to be and to do that of which they are capable. The good society, thus, involves ensuring people have access to that which is essential for the good life, not just for health. This access concerns nurses.

It is easy at this time—as in any other—for nurses to retreat into the ease of our usual duties of caring for the sick in hospitals, preventing illness in schools and primary care clinics, bringing babies into the world and caring for mothers, and conducting research to answer questions about how best to do all that. It is also easy to specialize—in critical care, in oncology and palliative care (my specialty), in pediatric and gerontologic care, and in psychiatric and mental health or community health nursing. Nurses' usual duties, which require specialized knowledge and skills, do indeed improve the health of individuals, families, and populations. But to stay only in these safe spaces fails to recognize the risk that supremacy of self-interest over the societal good, if unaddressed, will result in a worse society for ourselves and our patients. It also fails to recognize the power of nursing to bring about change. The central message of this book is that the profession of nursing is called to leave the comfort of and, indeed, to reach beyond narrowly defined nursing roles, whether clinical, administrative, or scientific, and address the ills of society that act as barriers to care—barriers to health care, yes, but also barriers to the kind of care that makes it possible for people to be and to do the best of which they are capable.

With more than twenty million registered nurses worldwide, nursing is the world's largest profession. It fascinates me when I go to a nursing conference and find nurses from the earth's four corners seeking the latest knowledge and skills so as to provide better patient care. Imagine nursing's power if nurses came from around the globe to learn how to address societal issues: the politics of war and violence; the economics of greed; the divisions of color and race, sex and gender; and the health of the planet upon which all life depends. Not studying war any longer would not only be an anthem of Africans brought in chains to the Americas; it could be nursing's anthem, if nursing would take a moral stance. War and health are opposites: one fractures; the other makes whole. Imagine if nurses worldwide came together with economists to address the economic well-being of the poor, such that no one fell short of the minimum income necessary for living a life in which they are able to be and do that of which they are capable. Imagine if nursing as a global profession came together with environmental scientists to bring about a stable climate, fertile soil for growing food that is safe to eat, and safe drinking water. Nursing has the power to do just that—to bring about the good society, to make the world a better place.

It was this power that motivated Nightingale. It motivated many of the historically important pioneers of the nursing profession who aimed for social reform. Lillian Wald, who lived as a nurse among poor immigrants in the tenements of New York City in the 1890s, focused her life's work on the relationship between nursing and the good society. In the 1960s, Florence Wald (no relation to Lillian) left her post as dean of the world's first university-based nursing school to bring the hospice movement to the United States. How society cares for the dying is a measure of its humanity. Florence Wald knew this, and she knew the power of nursing to improve the care of the dying and, thus, to improve society. These and countless other nurses have taught us that we must (in the language of ethics, we have an obligation to) address the societal ills of our time—to make the world a better place—through the power of nursing.

In 1867, the American poet Emma Lazarus penned a hagiographic poem about Nightingale. Then only in her late forties, Nightingale was already widely known and, as witnessed in Lazarus's stanzas, adored. In the poem, Lazarus portrays Nightingale as an angel "weeping o'er man's pain" and, in her weeping, an angel who works for a better world. This image appears again in Lazarus's 1883 poem, "The New Colossus," which she wrote for the pedestal of the Statue of Liberty in New York City's harbor, the harbor into which many immigrants came seeking a better world. I believe that Nightingale, the lady of the lamp, served as Lazarus's muse. In "The New Colossus," Lady Liberty gives rest to the tired, work to the poor, homes to the homeless, and peace to the tempest-tossed. She does this while lifting high her lamp, which sheds light on the promise of a good society, just as Nightingale's lamp symbolized hope for the hopeless. The image Lazarus portrays in "The New Colossus," I believe, is an image of a nurse who cares for the least among us, a nurse whose care brings the promise of the good society into the care-lessness of our (or, indeed, any) time.

I present this image in three parts. The first part presents the image of nursing as a moral profession. In Chapter 2, I argue that the profession's affirmation that humanity is the basis from which morality flows opens up nursing to being more than a health care profession. Because of the morality at its core, the profession of nursing is a human profession, one that is necessary for a good society. In Chapter 3, I suggest that, rather than human rights as the driver for the profession's work, the profession has obligations, which come before human rights. These obligations are to our common humanity. In the second part of the book, I describe six of these obligations that present an image of nursing as a full participant in bringing about a good society. These obligations are the obligation to work for equal opportunity to lead a good life, including—and for nursing especially—the opportunity to be able to lead a healthy life (Chapter 4); the obligation to provide assistance to those in need (Chapter 5); the obligations to promote peace (Chapter 6) and to provide safety (Chapter 7); the obligation to promote the health of Earth, upon which all human life depends (Chapter 8); and the obligation to have the confidence in the good that we do individually and collectively with our lives as nurses, that is, the obligation of respect (Chapter 9). Some people may argue for other obligations. I have chosen these six because I believe they apply universally—to all people in all times. Although they apply to all people, I believe that, when seen through the lens of nursing, they augur for a central role for the profession of nursing in bringing about a good society. In the final section, I present the good society as global, not only local or national, and the power of the profession of nursing to bring about the good society within the profession and in the world at large.

In my daily work as a university nursing professor, I encounter people who come into nursing as a second career. They come from all walks of life, many of them after having had successful careers in other fields. They come to nursing for the same reason that those two young men were content to be nurses in a rural village, the same reason Florence Wald cared for the dying, Lillian Wald lived and worked among the poor, and Nightingale founded the modern profession: they want to make the world a better place. As with Lazarus's poem, this is the image of nursing this book presents—and argues for. It is the image of a profession that ushers in a better world for all people.

Ushering in a better world for all people—the good society—begins with the basic belief that all people share one condition, one trait, from the moment we are born: we are human. It is the commonality of our humanity that I take up in the next chapter, a commonality that, I believe, grounds the good society.

PART I
NURSING IS A MORAL
PROFESSION

2

Nursing and Our
Common Humanity

In 1933, Raphael Lemkin, a Polish-Jewish lawyer, felt so incensed at the extermination of Armenians a decade earlier that he drafted a bill for the League of Nations to adopt as international law. The bill proclaimed that the extermination of a group of people who share a common ethnicity, race, religion, or other such collectivity is an offense "against the laws of nations." The principle upon which he based this offense was "the dignity of the individual." National interests, however, prevailed over concern for marginalized groups that were at risk of mass killings. The bill did not pass. Ten years later, Lemkin found himself in exile in the United States as the Nazis exterminated forty-nine members of his own family, along with six million more Jews, a quarter-million people with disabilities, and over two hundred thousand Roma, among many, many others. In 1943, as the Holocaust raged, Lemkin coined the term *genocide* in another legal attempt to face down the extermination of people simply because they belonged to a specific group. After the war, Lemkin continued his efforts to have genocide declared a crime under international law, and in 1948, the United Nations (UN), the postwar heir to the League of Nations, codified genocide as against international law. At the same time, the UN adopted the Universal Declaration of Human Rights. The declaration begins with the recognition of "the inherent dignity . . . of all members of the human family." Lemkin had forced the world to face "a problem from hell," to use the words of the human rights lawyer and former American diplomat Samantha Power, who has chronicled Lemkin's work.

Genocide had been declared illegal, and the basis of its illegality was that it is an offense against human dignity, which, at long last, the UN declared that all humans have. Human dignity is a permanent and essential characteristic that Lemkin's law against genocide aims to protect.

Not long after the UN Universal Declaration of Human Rights, the American Nurses Association's and the International Council of Nurses' codes of ethics adopted the same premises, namely, that inherent in nursing practice is respect for human dignity, and that it is from this dignity that the profession's morality flows.

However fundamental the concept of dignity is—and surely it is—its precise definition is slippery, and in philosophy it can be a dangerous tool. Some philosophers, such as John Rawls, thought it too undefined to serve a foundational role in his philosophy of justice. A contemporary philosopher, Simon Blackburn, does not even mention it in his justly famous introduction to ethics. Another contemporary philosopher, Peter Singer, argues that dignity does not allow for quality of life. For example, some people argue that clinician-assisted death allows for the recognition that one's quality of life has deteriorated to the point at which life is not worth living. They invoke dignity to justify clinician-assisted death, arguing that it preserves dignity, while even others say that clinician-assisted death militates against dignity. The concept of dignity can be made to carry with it overtones of elitism (dignity as conferred by status or role) or be based in religious belief (dignity because humans are made in the image of God). Indeed, some people, such as the contemporary psychologist Steven Pinker, think that the concept is used by some to impose religious belief on others' morality. This squishiness notwithstanding, Lemkin, the UN delegates who adopted the declaration, and the nurses who wrote and adopted the profession's ethics codes used dignity as the concept that expresses the value of every human being.

The good society begins with dignity, for one of the demands of human dignity is that all humans are viewed and treated equally.

In the early 1970s, my wife was a young girl traveling from her home in Gaborone, Botswana, to the international airport in Johannesburg, South Africa, with her family and one of Botswana's elder statesmen. Botswana was then—and is now—a democracy in which all people were treated equally by law, regardless of color. It shared a border with South Africa. In the 1970s, South Africa was a nondemocratic country ruled under the apartheid system. Apartheid segregated people of color from white people, and it did not allow people of color to elect the officials who ran the country's government. It seems simplistic to say—simplistic in the sense that its obvious wrongness still shocks—that the apartheid system treated people of color as unequal to white people; but it was not at all a simple matter. Once my wife, her family, and this elder statesman crossed into South Africa and drew near the airport, they stopped at a roadside café to get a drink, use the facilities, and tidy up before checking in at the gate. It had been a long, hot, and dusty journey. But the elder statesman, being black, could not go into the café, nor could he use the café's facilities. They were reserved for whites only. To this day, my wife recalls the shame she felt at hearing the white café manager tell a man the people of Botswana revered that he had to use the bush—the weeds outside—as his toilet. How could a person who was so esteemed in one country become her unequal merely by crossing into another country? Of course, a person does not become unequal to other people by crossing into another country. But the then–South African regime and the people that propped it up treated people of color as if they were lesser.

The same was true in many states in the United States until 1964, when the Civil Rights Act outlawed discrimination based on race, color, religion, sex, or national origin. People of color who faced apartheid conditions in the United States could cross the border into Canada and not face them. By stepping over a political—and imaginary—line (it is not a line drawn into the foundations of the earth), did they become different?

The seventeenth-century philosopher John Locke understood the shame of people being treated as lesser than others. In Locke's time, monarchs ruled Europe with absolute authority, and they topped a social hierarchy that, as one moved down it, considered people less and less important. People higher up the social hierarchy could, with impunity, treat people lower down the social hierarchy with disdain and, sometimes, brutality. This inequality, and the mistreatment of others it permitted, incensed Locke to the point that he argued against it, not a fashionable thing to do in his time. He had to flee his native England because of what he argued. His argument, essentially, was that, when the hierarchy was stripped away and people stood before each other as they are in "a state of nature," all people are the same. One way of thinking about this is that, in the earliest of times, before hierarchies were imposed on society, humans stood before each other equally. Yet another way of thinking about it is that, when societal façades are stripped away and we get down to the kernel of truth about who we are, we are all the same. That is, in the state of nature when we first come out of our mothers' wombs, we are equal. In our natural state, we share equality. That equality is our common humanity. This common humanity is the moral basis of our relationship with each other. It is the moral truth that holds a good society together.

My wife—as a young girl, before she had much by way of moral education—knew this. Perhaps she, as a child, lived more in a state of nature than the white South African regime that imposed the apartheid system. In the end, the apartheid system fell, and what my wife knew was right came about. South Africa became a democratic country in 1994, and when it did, it enshrined in its new constitution what Locke said is naturally the case: all humans are equal. The South African constitution states that the country is founded on the value of "human dignity" and "the achievement of equality." Now in South Africa, a black person, whether a revered elder statesperson or a young child, is equal to a white person. There is but one humanity. This too is what Lemkin's international law against genocide and the UN declaration enshrined: we have a common—that is, we all have an equal share in—humanity.

This, of course, is at the heart of nursing practice. We treat every person the same. When we see someone who needs nursing care and we are able to give it, we must do so, no matter who the person is. It is essential as nurses that we believe in the equality of humanity. What we would do for one person as a nurse is what we would do for any other person in the same situation. It is in this way that the basis of nursing practice counters the care-lessness of this or of any time: against the forces that seek to divide humanity—Nazism, racism, nationalism, and all other "isms" that proclaim that we should not care for a people group—nursing proclaims that we care for all people, regardless of who they are, for in the state of nature, we are all the same.

This equal treatment is the respect that we show our common humanity. The word *respect*, in its Latin origins, means to look back at. When we respect others, when we care for all people equally, it is as if we stand outside ourselves and look back upon our and others' humanity and recognize it. I have had this experience when I least expected it.

I was abroad doing palliative care research. I walked into the room of a man in his midtwenties who was dying of a rare cancer. It had eaten away a good portion of his right femur and had spread to his skin. He was in great pain; it was hard to manage it. The stench from his rotting flesh overwhelmed me. I had to set aside my revulsion and go into my professional mode. I approached his care scientifically: How much morphine could I safely give him? Could I use metronidazole to reduce the foul odor? I tried to calculate his prognosis—how long did he have to endure this suffering? I sat down near him, his face drawn and eyes bloodshot. He looked directly at me. Neither of us uttered a word. We just looked at each other, he from his deathbed and me in my white lab coat with my stethoscope draped around my neck. In that moment, something changed. I thought that I could see myself in him, as if looking in a mirror. It seemed to me that he too saw himself in me, although there was no way of knowing if this was true. Despite our different conditions (he was dying, I was well) and our positions (he was a patient, I was a nurse), we were both just human. Perhaps many of you have experienced this moment—this kind of mystical moment—when you looked at someone and saw yourself in that person. That day, I saw my own humanity in his. Through respect for our shared humanity, I recognized our bond.

Crimes against humanity, such as genocide and the crimes perpetrated within apartheid systems, are crimes that arise from disrespecting humanity. The perpetrators of these crimes fail to see themselves in those against whom they commit crimes; they fail to see the humanity they share with their own victims. In so doing, they disrespect—and thus deny—their own humanity. Their crimes are crimes against humanity—against the victims' humanity but also against the perpetrators' humanity. In effect, the perpetrators deny their own participation in humanity.

However, when we, as nurses, look back upon ourselves in others while caring for them, we acknowledge and respect our shared humanity. We care for them as we would care for all humans, including ourselves.

Writing after Locke, the eighteenth-century German philosopher Immanuel Kant called this respect the categorical imperative. The categorical imperative is an unconditional moral obligation that never changes over time or according to circumstance. The categorical imperative means that we should act toward ourselves and other people in ways that apply universally; that is, we should act toward ourselves and other people in ways that would be good even if the times and the circumstances were different.

Nursing practice embodies the categorical imperative, because it treats everyone the same, as a human worthy of care. I believe that when we say to ourselves, "Well, if I were this patient . . .," we are, in fact, giving voice to the experience I called a kind of mystical experience in which we see our own humanity in the patient. This is why human dignity is inherent in nursing practice: because nursing practice respects the common humanity of nurse and of patient.

Of course, throughout the modern history of nursing there have been nurses who have perpetrated crimes against humanity. Contemporary nurse scholars Susan Benedict and Linda Shields have chronicled such crimes committed by nurses and midwives during the Holocaust. Nurses also participated in the crimes of apartheid. These nurses disrespected humanity—the humanity in others but also, because humanity is equally shared, the humanity in themselves. And yet, there have been nurses who, in peril of their own lives, have respected the common humanity in these situations: non-Jewish nurses during the Holocaust and white nurses during apartheid who rescued Jews and who treated people of color as they would treat anyone. These nurses acted in ways that could be universally applied, and in so doing, they respected the humanity in themselves and others. This is why, often, when people do heroic deeds, such as these nurses, they often decry being called heroes. They say they did what they would have wanted others to do for them if their roles were reversed. It is what a human does for humans.

This is what I believe is meant by human dignity: our common humanity. And when we see this, we will also see that from our common humanity arise common obligations.

3

Nursing and Obligation

I do not know of a more idealistic age than nine. Nine-year-old children want to do good—and they think they can. Nine-year-old children are old enough to notice injustices, and yet they are not old enough to believe that injustices cannot be addressed or that their solutions are not just fantasies. When my son was nine, he became aware of the poor people around him. He said there should not be money so that there would not be any poor people. Ten years later, some economists think that eliminating cash would be an important step in creating a more equitable economy. When I was nine, I wanted to help a man who could not use his legs.

Growing up, my family and I lived only about an hour's drive north of the US-Mexico border. My parents' good friends lived in the Mexican border town that was nearest us, San Luis Río Colorado. Mr. and Mrs. Garcia—or Señor y Señora Garcia, as we called them—had two boys: Juanito, who was about a year younger than me, and Jacob, who was a baby when I was nine. I know this because that year, at my behest, my parents drove me to San Luis and dropped me off to spend the summer with the Garcias.

Due to the poor Mexican economy at the time, Señor Garcia could not find work in San Luis. The town straddled the Colorado River, the same river that ran within a few miles of my home upstream. Upstream, the river irrigated the fertile diluvian soils of the Colorado River valley. Before modern damming, spring floods brought Rocky Mountain soil downstream to the valley, where farmers grew produce. Señor Garcia regaled me with stories about the river in Mexico, the river before the upstream dams and before the United States used its waters to quench its desert cities' voracious thirst. When he was a boy, he said, it flowed like a torrent into the Gulf of California, locally known as Mar de Cortés. Farmers in San Luis, and other Mexican border towns, irrigated their farms with it, just as my family did in the United States. But then the United States built the dams that created large reservoirs for its desert cities: Los Angeles, Las Vegas, and Phoenix. And farmers in the United States started using chemicals. These farmers would spread fertilizers, pesticides, and herbicides; irrigate the land; and then return the run-off water, now awash with these chemicals, back into the river downstream, just before the Mexican border. By the time the river water got to San Luis, all that was left was a trickle of pure pollution. Señor Garcia had been a farmer on his own land, land that was no longer viable due to lack of clean irrigation water. He could not find work in Mexico, and so daily, he would sneak into the United States, crawling under fences or wading through the river's unclean waters, to work as a day laborer on US farms upstream where the abundant water was clean. Señora Garcia ran the affairs of the house and was active in her church.

That summer was hot and, unlike my family home just sixty miles north, the Garcias' home did not have air conditioning. On those long summer days, Jacob crawled along the house's bare cement floors, while Juanito and I played soccer in the backyard, an all-dirt pitch. We played barefoot. Sometimes, Señora Garcia would come out to our pitch and tell us to go to the store to get what she needed for cooking. Sugar, flour, lard, beans—these are the ingredients I remember most. Vegetables came from their expansive garden that was at the back of our pitch. It was an oasis plopped down amid the desert sands, watered by a well Señor Garcia had dug deep into the clean waters of an aquifer. Señor Garcia had made it clear—in frightening terms—that the garden was off limits. But I was not that good with my aim. I remember furtively glancing at the house when I would mistakenly kick the ball into that Eden.

On the way to the store, Juanito and I always passed an old man who perched himself on a corner of a busy intersection. He asked the passersby, all of whom he seemed to know by name, for money. Something was wrong with his legs. They looked thin, and when I once saw him try to move, I realized they did not work. They flopped around. He "ambulated" by dragging himself by his hands—crawling like Jacob but without moving his knees in co-ordination with his arms. An old man with gray hair and a sun-parched face crawling around like a baby: I felt the wrong—the horror—of it, and my nine-year-old heart wanted to fix it. I wanted to give this man the ability to get around, and I wanted to give him lots of money. I wanted to make his world better.

When I would get back to the Garcias' home after these errands, I would kick the ball around and daydream about giving money to everyone who needed it. I was not as smart as my son, per-haps, to realize that money is a source of the problem, but I did see that inequalities were real and were greater problems for people who had vulnerabilities. I would daydream that that man had a wheelchair. I would daydream that he had a home and that I had helped my dad build a ramp up to the front door. I could see my-self driving nails into the planks of that ramp as they ran up to his air-conditioned home.

I would also daydream about fixing the Colorado River. Mexicans, after all, deserved clean water for farming and drinking as much as we did. Their humanity was the same as ours—the same as everybody's. Little did I know that water would motivate poli-tics, within and outside my country, and that the people who were motivated by water cared less about the poor and vulnerable and more about their self-interests—the interests of the rich and pow-erful. But when one approaches the problem from the point of view of a nine-year-old boy, does it not make sense that we who live up-stream owe clean water to people who live downstream? Is it not our obligation to be good stewards of the water we have access to? Is it not our obligation to treat the people downstream as we would want to be treated ourselves?

I do not believe now, as a grown man, that my nine-year-old daydreams were merely quixotic. I believe they derived from a drive within to feel—and to want to respond to—the vulnerabilities of others. Witness babies who begin to cry when they hear other babies cry: it is human to feel with—and to respond to—others. I now believe that my desire to do something for this man—my desire to respect his humanity—was the basis of obligation. I also believe that this desire originated in the long history of human development in which we have learned over thousands and thousands of years that we are more likely to survive if we help others in the way we would want anyone, including ourselves, to be helped. I had an obligation to that man: to help him. But I also had an obligation to myself, for by helping him I would be furthering my own cause: I would be respecting my own humanity as I respected his. By helping him, I would make the world just that much better. A better world for him, after all, is better for me too.

This was an awakening experience. Perhaps it was the first time I was able to imagine myself in someone else's plight. Maybe it was the first time I could look back upon myself by looking at him, and in so doing, maybe it was the first time I became aware of my own vulnerability. Perhaps I wanted to do something about the old man's plight for my own sake: so I did not feel so vulnerable myself.

Alongside the impulse to respond to others' needs sits the impulse to protect oneself. With this impulse, we can turn inward with fear, bumping up our shoulder in the face of someone who appears threatening, putting our hands over our wounds when someone tries to clean them, not sharing with others when we fear we will not have enough for ourselves. This self-interest impulse is as deep—as primordial—as the impulse to feel with, and respond to, others. These two impulses are intertwined, not competing. We have these awakening moments in our lives when we are aware that these two impulses—the other-oriented impulse and the self-interest impulse—complement: I protect myself by helping others.

In other words, my obligation to myself, my obligation to the old man perched on the street corner, and my obligation to Señor Garcia's need for clean water were all the same. In my nine-year-old mind, I knew that I owed it to others and to myself to do something about others' plight. My nine-year-old mind comprehended—indeed, respected—our common humanity.

"Obligation" is an old word. Some may even think of it as a quaint word. I remember my grandfather replying to people who performed good deeds on his behalf with, "I am much obliged." In that use, the word carries with it a sense of debt. My grandfather owed a debt of gratitude to the people who did something good for him. That old meaning of being in debt to someone is precisely what I mean by "obligation." As I shall explain later, I owed a debt to the old man and to Señor Garcia. I owed a debt to our common humanity.

Cicero, the Roman philosopher who wrote in the first century before the Common Era, thought that the greatest debt—the greatest obligation—we have is to virtue itself. We repay this debt by being honest, prudent, fair, temperate, and courageous. That is, we repay our debt to virtue by developing in ourselves virtuous habits. Habits are an outward sign of inward devotions. We cultivate habits in ourselves over time to show forth our inward devotions. It may be tempting to tell a "harmless lie," a "social, polite lie," such as telling a friend who invites you to a party that you have another commitment when, in fact, you just do not want to go. But such a lie would stand in opposition to our inward devotion to the virtue, truth, to which we owe a debt. If you do not pay your debt to truth, your debt will grow, and eventually the habit of telling lies will make you an untrustworthy person. In this way, we cannot escape obligations. Unless we fulfill them, they remain outstanding debts.

In addition to our obligation to virtue itself, Cicero thought that we have certain obligations that arise out of the roles we have in life, of which he said we have four. First, we all have the role of being rational. It is in this role that we assess how well we fulfill our obligations; that is, we owe a debt to ourselves to judge how faithful we have been to our obligations. Second, we have individual natural talents and abilities; we are good at some things and not at others. We cannot fight against what we are good at or try to mimic others to achieve what they have achieved. Rather, we owe a debt to ourselves to know what we are good at and work hardest at doing it, for it is by doing what we are good at that we will make great personal contributions. Third, we all play a role we have not chosen. We are born into families. We are sons and daughters, sisters and brothers. We have an obligation to be good in these roles, which are beyond our control. The fourth role is the role we have chosen. It is that to which we have decided to devote our lives. In this role, we choose the kind of person we wish to be and the kind of life we wish to live. When we do, we owe a debt to ourselves—and to others who depend upon us in that role—to do it well. In this role, the role we have chosen, we find the fullest expression of the debt we owe to humanity—to the humanity we share with others past, present, and future, the common humanity.

You have chosen to be a nurse—or maybe you are thinking about becoming a nurse. Maybe you have been touched by a nurse and you want to understand what drove him or her to provide such life-changing care for you. That nurse was devoted to nursing, and in that devotion, he or she was faithful to the debt he or she owed you—the debt he or she owed the humanity you both shared—by virtue of choosing to become a nurse.

Nursing is a health care profession, and as such, it demands that we practice competently, for, as with all health care professions, we have the privilege of holding people's lives in our hands. We can move beyond being competent nurses to become expert nurses, and we can, over the course of our careers, draw upon the latest nursing science to improve our expertise. Nursing, practiced this way, is a highly technical endeavor focused on providing the latest scientifically based interventions to restore or promote patients' health or to enable them to have a good death. This approach to nursing—technical and scientific—would not be wrong, but it would not embody the fullness of the privilege of the profession. That privilege is to choose to nurse others to health or to a peaceful death because, in so doing, one respects humanity. And by respecting humanity, one makes the world a better place.

Nursing is at a crossroads about the degree to which it looks to science to define it as a profession. People from many fields, not just nursing, have turned to science to "change and improve the world." To these people, science can "solve some of the most pressing issues of our times," including teaching us how "to live sustainably." Life sciences, they proclaim, "save lives," and technology will "allow us to pursue solutions we never would have dreamed possible even a decade ago." Science may give us insight into the way the world works, but science cannot teach us how to live sustainably. Nor can science solve all of the pressing issues that affect people's lives—issues of political unrest, war, and violence; the threat of nuclear war and in general the arms trade; climate change; poverty, hunger, clean water, and safe food; and lack of education. Science can, of course, help. But the most expedient and effective solutions to many of life's most pressing problems concern human behavior—how we live with each other in the world. Moreover, science will not save lives, nor could it ever. Science may extend life. It has offered us vaccines. The old man whose legs did not work likely had had polio. Today, with the polio vaccine, there are indeed fewer people with nonworking legs. Science may one day find a cure for cancer, but even then, science will only delay death, for all people die. That is the human condition. Paradoxically, as agricultural chemical technologies contributed solutions to some problems thought intractable a generation ago, we now recognize that these solutions have contributed to people's untimely deaths from cancer and to the earth's degradation, as Señor Garcia knew forty years ago. And global climate change is in part driven by the long-term effects of human uses of the scientific technologies of the industrial age. Science alone cannot change or improve the world, but how we live can.

Nursing science has advanced our understanding of how to keep people healthy, how to care for the sick in ways that restore health, and how to enable peaceful deaths. Nursing science is instrumental; it helps us to better discharge our duties. But nursing involves working with people: humans working with humans. As such, it involves the humanities as much as it involves science. When we think of nursing as a humanity, we then see science's place in nursing. Science is inert: it is not human; it does not care. Nurses care. The endeavor of nursing is one in which we who are nurses seek to faithfully discharge our obligations, obligations that become ours by virtue of having chosen to be nurses. And when we faithfully discharge our nursing obligations, we ultimately make the world a better place.

When one looks at nursing in this way—that is, when one chooses to perform one's work as a nurse because that work is about bettering the world—nursing becomes a calling. A calling is work that the world needs to have done. But it also brings satisfaction to the doer. The twentieth-century nurse-theorist Virginia Henderson remarked that excellent nurses do not work to impress others; rather, they work "*solely* for the inner satisfaction of knowing they have helped one human being after another." This is where obligation and calling intersect: when a person undertakes the work of nursing in the service of our common humanity—that is, out of a sense of obligation toward humanity—this work begets in one a sense of satisfaction. In addition, as we nurses make the world a better place through acts of caring for individuals, we make the world a better place for all, including ourselves.

When what I do betters the world for you and me, together we share in the benefits of a better world. However, when I look at my world-bettering work as an obligation, not only do we share in the benefits of that work, but also my work becomes a kind of repayment of my debt. I am obliged to you for the benefits that come to me through my work done on your behalf. At the same time, I call upon you to share in this debt, a debt you owe for the benefits accrued to you. When we acknowledge this mutual debt and seek to repay each other, we have a social contract that arises from our discharging our debts to our shared humanity. Nursing then becomes part of the bond of society. By caring, we call on others—even those for whom we have not cared—to respect our common humanity. We call on them to feel obliged to care about making the world a better place. The work of nursing calls society to its obligations.

The choice to become a nurse necessarily involves taking a particular position in society, a position that carries with it a contract to care.

The modern history of nursing is punctuated with nurses working to improve society and calling others, in their time and we who live long after their time, to respond in like measure. In the nineteenth century, Florence Nightingale worked to improve hospital-based treatment, public sanitation for the world's poor, income inequality, and working conditions; and she called upon others, particularly lawmakers, to do the same. Fifteen years after the American Civil War, Clara Barton, at sixty years of age, went to Europe to learn about a budding movement there to provide relief to people wounded by war. She extended that movement to the United States by founding the American Red Cross, which now calls upon people around the world to improve the lives of others. Around the same time, Dorothea Dix advocated on behalf of the mentally ill. Through her efforts, some of the first publicly funded institutions for people who had mental illness were created. In the late nineteenth and early twentieth centuries, Mary Mahoney, the first African American in the United States to train and work as a professional nurse, addressed racial inequalities and, through her work on voting, called others to address suffrage and other civil liberties deprived from people because of the color of their skin, the sex of their birth, or their gender. In the 1920s, Margaret Sanger founded the American Birth Control League, which later became Planned Parenthood. In the 1960s, Florence Wald, who brought the hospice movement to the United States, called lawmakers to make hospice a Medicare benefit so that the Unites States would be a society that provides for its dying the conditions necessary for peaceful deaths. These nurses, and many more throughout nursing history, answered the call—the obligation—to improve society, and they called others, especially non-nurses, to join in that obligation.

It is fashionable in nursing to rest the ethical behavior of nurses on promoting, advocating, and protecting the rights of patients, rights that, some say, arise out of human dignity, rather than on fulfilling obligations toward our common humanity. From this fashion has come campaigns for patients' bills of rights. "Rights" is common political language, especially in the United States; we are comfortable with it. And admittedly, work done on behalf of ensuring that all people have equal access to quality health care is important. But to base our health care ethics on rights leads to an insuperable problem. A person may be disenfranchised from a right but may be unable to do anything about it. Consider people who, as you read these words, do not have access to quality health care because of where they live, because of their lack of employment or poor socioeconomic status, or because of past medical history—for whatever reason. We can say that they have a right to health care. We can also say that this right is based on the fundamental right of human dignity, and indeed it is, as the UN Universal Declaration of Human Rights proclaims. But how are the people who do not have access to quality health care to ensure their right to it? If they are unable to ensure their rights, then who is?

Some may argue that the old man I met in Mexico when I was nine years old was active in promoting his rights by begging on the street corner. He was, after all, asking for people to give him money, and by giving him money, people would be addressing his rights, if only in a temporary way. Even if we say he was active in promoting his rights, he was only active by agitating for others to act on his behalf. And yet, how many passersby did not act on his behalf, or merely threw a few centavos his way? How many passersby turned their faces in a self-protective move? *I have to feed my own family. I don't have enough money to spare for that old man.* Think about Señor Garcia too. How was he to ensure his right to a Colorado River that reached Mexico with enough clean water for farming? How was I to ensure it? How was the Mexican government to ensure it against the Goliath of the US government? When it comes to what we call welfare rights, that is, rights to the things people need to have adequate health and well-being, it is easy to think that we do not need to act at all. Does not someone else—the government, or the good people at Oxfam—bear the responsibility to act on behalf of others' rights to food, shelter, clean water, and the means to provide for one's family? We all have rights, but the problem with rights is, who is to ensure them?

Rights are easier to talk about than obligations. Rights are more contained, and they are less frightening to deal with, perhaps because they distance us from those who are not enfranchised with them. Our talk becomes about rights, not about what we owe our fellow humans. We can say that someone has a right to quality health care, but saying that does not force us into action. We can remain passive in deed while active in speech. Obligations, on the other hand, require us to act. Even the old man who had perched himself on the street corner to seek donations from people so that he had the means to supply for his welfare had rights; yet these rights did not matter unless someone felt obligated to act. And what, exactly, were others' obligations toward him? Just to give him money? When we talk about this old man's rights—or any rights, for that matter—we only talk about "the less powerful part" of the issue, the contemporary British philosopher Onora O'Neill says. The more powerful part is our obligations.

Simone Weil, a French philosopher and political activist who wrote during World War II, recognized an important difference between rights and obligations. Rights, she said, are meaningless without the context of others around you, others with obligations that compel them to act toward you in certain ways. That is, rights start with others' obligations. Obligations, however, always start with you. Because of this difference, Weil said that "the notion of obligations comes before the notion of rights."

This is what happened with me in my experience with the old man. I felt an awareness that I had an obligation to him—indeed, an obligation toward our common humanity. I felt obligated to act on his behalf, out of respect for our common humanity. My obligations toward him, however, were prior to any rights he may have had. I would have accorded him rights only when I acted upon my obligations toward him. And my actions on his behalf—actions that would have accorded him rights—would have been taken in the context of the conditions of his life. He was disabled, and he sought sustenance through asking others for money. Compared to him, I was able-bodied, and my parents, though not rich by US standards, could supply for my needs. The welfare rights that the old man had were embedded in his not fully having them, at least not when compared to my welfare. His rights, that is, were relative to the facts of his existence. In this way, rights are always relative to the context of our lives.

Obligations, however, are universal. They are not conditioned by the facts of our lives, the facts that condition the different rights we have at different times and in different circumstances of our lives. Obligations, unlike rights, are above the facts of our lives. They are, to use Weil's word, "eternal." Though eternal, obligations have a real effect on how we ought to behave in our daily lives. I have spent a good deal of my career exploring how that which is universal (or to use Weil's language, how that which is eternal) ought to affect how we choose to live. No concept is more profound and yet has more of a daily impact on how we ought to live than the concept of obligations.

Any nursing theory—whether about nursing ethics or about nursing science that focuses not just on theory but also on caring for people—begins with obligations. If nursing science tells us that a certain intervention will help to promote or restore health for some people, or that it will help some people to have more peaceful deaths, then we are obligated to do it for those people. But nursing science traffics in the specific. That is the nature of science. For science to propose a solution to a clinical problem, the problem must be narrowly defined. But the problems that confront nursing as a profession—the problems that prevent people around the world from enjoying the conditions necessary for health—are global in scale. We will only fully confront these problems when we focus on nursing's universal obligations toward our common humanity. It is not that these obligations are only shared by nurses. To be sure, the whole of the human community shares in them; they are universal obligations. But I contend that nursing cannot be the profession it says it is—a profession that promotes and restores health and provides for peaceful deaths—without fulfilling certain obligations toward our common humanity. And I contend that, when nursing acts on these obligations, the world becomes a better place.

Let us now turn to six of these obligations—equality, assistance, peace, safety, Earth, and respect—and think about how, in fulfilling them, nurses, and the profession, contribute to making the world a better place.

PART II
THE OBLIGATIONS
OF NURSING

4

Equality

The Garcias may not have had as much money as my family. Their house had bare cement floors, had no air conditioning, and sat on a dirt road. But we both bought the food we needed at grocery stores, and we both supplemented that food with produce from verdant vegetable gardens that our parents tended. The children of both our families went to school and had summers off for leisure; on both sides of the border, the era of children laboring in the fields for the harvest had long since passed. I knew that Señor Garcia had tough working conditions, but I saw him as a strong, strapping man who provided for his family, the same as my father. To my nine-year-old eyes, we were pretty much equal. The inequalities that existed—and there were inequalities—were imperceptible to me at that age. But even at that age, I recognized the inequality between me and the man who begged for money on the street corner in San Luis, Mexico. Even as a young boy, I knew that, compared to me, he was poor. I also knew that, compared to him, the Garcias and my family were well off. My nine-year-old mind and heart could take that in. I was aware of the inequalities that separated him from us. I felt the shame of it, the embarrassment that came from my saying to him, "I'm sorry, sir. All I can give you is a few cents."

Why should inequality concern us? Is not inequality just the way things are? My brothers are taller and stronger than me, which means that, in matters of brute force, I am always their unequal. Moreover, are not some people born with natural talents that most of us could only wish for? I know of people who spent many years practicing the piano, striving to be good, but were never as good as people born with the gift. Prodigies, as we call them, are unequal to us mere mortals. In the ranks of naturally gifted pianists, there are few. Some aspects of heredity (height, for example) and natural talent are legitimate differences among people.

In addition, there are legitimate differences that arise from the choices people make for themselves. Monks all over the world and in various religions choose to be poor. Some, in fact, choose to be beggars. I have witnessed Theravada Buddhist monks engage in the ancient practice of going into the community every morning with their begging bowls and entreating passersby to give them food. The monks value this begging way of life, as it serves the greater purpose of calling the community to charitable acts. But most important, they are capable of leading this way of life. Even though they are unequal to the community in some ways, they are free to be and to do that of which they are capable. As I mentioned in Chapter 1, Amartya Sen says the good society gives individuals this freedom. Everyone having this freedom, says Sen, is the essence of equality. Essentially, equality is the freedom to choose the way of life one has reason to value.

When we evaluate others' lives through the lens of equality, we begin by considering what people are able to be and to do, which the contemporary philosopher Martha Nussbaum calls capacities. Nussbaum lists ten essential capacities that all societies, to be good societies, should nourish equally for all people. When in nursing we speak of equality, what we mean is equality in the distribution of these essential capacities.

In Nussbaum's list is bodily integrity (that is, the ability to change locations freely and to have sovereignty over one's body). When as a boy I saw the man whose legs did not work, his begging did not strike me as odd. I had seen begging before, and of course, as a child I had begged—or at the very least, pleaded—for something I wanted but did not have other means of getting. But I had not seen someone whose bodily integrity was so impaired. Upon looking at him, I knew that I would not want to be like him. I knew I would not want to get around by crawling. I remember his elbows and hands looking deformed from the calluses that had developed from his dragging himself about. It was his lack of bodily integrity—his inability to change locations in a way that did not imperil his health and well-being—that struck me. How could he live a good life—a life in which he had the capacity to flourish—in the state he was in? He lacked a capacity fundamental to the possibility of having a life he—indeed, any member of society—had reason to value.

It is for this reason that societies have enacted laws that require accessible public accommodations, commercial facilities, transportation, and telecommunications: so that people with physical disabilities have the same capacity to flourish—the same capacity to have a good life—as anyone else. And that is what is at stake, still, in my memory of the man whose legs did not work. When the effects of heredity and natural talent are controlled for, in my memory, that man and I had unequal capacities to flourish. That is morally wrong.

Morally wrong inequality gives some people an advantage over others when it comes to the capacities necessary to flourish—that is, the capacities necessary to have a good life. Indeed, this asymmetry defines immoral inequality. To be moral, the man and I needed to be symmetrical in our possession of these capacities. He was not able to change locations freely, but I was. He needed an assistive device, and public spaces needed to be accessible to him while using this device. Our asymmetrical capacity needed to be evened out by a society that valued him as much as it valued me.

I felt this asymmetry. It is a feeling that I have not, these many years later, forgotten. It arises out of the wrongness of his situation. It is the feeling that goes with Kant's categorical imperative, which I mentioned in Chapter 2: I could not wish his situation to be universal. Indeed, if his situation were mine, my ability to lead a good life would be unequal to most other people. It would be easy to pervert this feeling into horror, looking at him and seeing how awful his life is and saying how thankful I am that I do not have his life, because, if I did, it would be horrible. That "How horrible!" feeling is akin to the voyeur who looks upon people who are disadvantaged and says, "Look at how good my life is compared with theirs." It turns the focus away from how inequality is a state we can work to correct and onto seeing people who experience inequality as freaks in life's show, a human who is less than human and upon whom the voyeur looks for his or her interest. In so doing, the voyeur has disrespected his own humanity.

To be motivated to work for equality, we must think that we too share humanity with those who experience inequalities. That is, we must believe that there ought to be symmetry among all people in the capacities necessary for the good life. This belief should transform the emotion we feel when we see people who do not have equal capacities to flourish, from one that leads to inaction ("How horrible!") to one that compels us to work for equality ("We both are humans!").

When nurses care for others in ways that promote equal capacities, nursing promotes the good society. As nurses, we are the ambulation of those who cannot walk, the sight of the blind, the calm assurance of first-time parents, the knowledge of how to change lifestyle to manage heart disease and type 2 diabetes, until our patients gain independence and can do those things for themselves. We raise our patients' capacities, not by bringing our- selves down to their level of incapacity but by extending to them the capacities for flourishing, and thus, for leading a good life until they can develop these capacities for themselves. When asymmetry exists, nursing seeks to even it out.

One may counter that this view of nursing's work is a coloni- alist, or hegemonic, view. Perhaps someone, for some reason, might value crawling on hands and elbows. Maybe this person believes, for instance, that suffering is redemptive. But surely, not even this person would require that of others. Surely, this person would accept that, for humans to live their lives in such a way that their capacities to lead a good life are not restricted, they need to be able to get around on their own.

Suppose the man could not use his legs because he had had polio as a child. Suppose that he was born not long after Jonas Salk's polio vaccine became widely available. However, by accident of where he was born and lived, he did not have access to the vaccine. This lack of access changed his capacities for physical health and bodily integrity in ways that people who received the vaccine would never experience. His lack of access made him unequal to the people who had been vaccinated. This unequal access to the vaccine is morally significant because it changed his capacities. Moreover, if he did not have access to the vaccine and others did, even before he contracted polio when he still had bodily integrity and physical health, he was unequal to people who had access to the vaccine: they would never have been exposed to the possibility of their bodily diminution as he was.

Given what had happened to him, and the physical condition he had to live with, he still could have achieved the condition necessary for better health with the right assistance. One of nursing's tenets is that all people, regardless of their bodily integrity, can achieve better health. I do not mean simple physical health, that is, a disease-free state. Rather, I mean the lived experience of health beyond medical definition. I have been a nurse for patients who, though they were dying, had a sense of health. They had recreated their identities amid life-limiting diseases, and thus, they had come to a sense of health that was beyond disease. They had emotionally and spiritually conquered disease. According to the twentieth-century theologian Paul Tillich, the capacity to conquer disease psychologically, socially, and spiritually is the capacity for health, for to be alive is to live with the possibility—indeed, the reality—of disease and eventual death. But having the capacity to conquer disease, even though we may not cure it, is having the capacity for health. Nursing seeks to bring that capacity to all people. And for the profession of nursing, the greatest inequality is an asymmetry in people's capacity for health.

The capacity for health—for conquering disease—is not only an internal capacity. It is also economic. The epidemiologists Richard Wilkinson and Kate Pickett, in their 2009 book *The Spirit Level: Why Greater Equality Makes Societies Stronger*, used international and state-level data from the United States to look at the association between income inequality and health outcomes. They found that societies with greater income inequality have a greater prevalence of mental illness, more drug use, higher infant mortality and teenage pregnancy rates, and more obese adults than societies in which income was more equal. They also found that more unequal societies have higher homicide and imprisonment rates. Children experience more conflict and more of them drop out of high school. Income inequality ought to concern nurses as a profession, as it creates inequality in the capacity to conquer disease.

Elizabeth Bradley and her colleagues at the Yale School of Public Health used state-level and national data from the United States to look at the association between health outcomes and the ratio of government expenditure on social services and public health to expenditure on health care. They found that states with a higher ratio of spending on social services and public health to spending on health care had significantly better health outcomes one and two years later. These better health outcomes were fewer adults who had obesity and who had asthma, fewer "mentally unhealthy" days, fewer days with activity limitations, and lower rates of death from lung cancer, acute myocardial infarction, and type 2 diabetes. Bradley and her coauthors concluded that, when we think about health care spending, we should also think about investment in social services and public health. This makes sense, for spending on social services and public health is one way to even out the societal inequalities that create inequality in the capacity to conquer disease, inequalities in income, education, the physical environment, employment, social support networks, and access to quality health care, especially preventive health care. In other words, spending on social services and public health helps to even out the capacity for conquering disease. As Bradley and colleagues' work shows, the conditions necessary for psychological, social, and spiritual health are necessary for physical health, rather than the other way around. It is for this reason that nursing has long been interested in the equality of the conditions necessary for a good life.

Jessie Beard, a nurse writing in the *American Journal of Nursing* in 1917, knew the truth of what Wilkinson and Pickett and Bradley and colleagues found a hundred years later. Nurses encounter patients' economic and social realities either at the bedside or in their homes. The profession of nursing is concerned with these realities, Beard says. In her opinion, nurses seek to improve patients' economic and social conditions so that they do not need our nursing care, for, as we now know empirically, the capacities necessary for a good life play a part in health. Even before Beard, Lillian Wald established public health nursing in the squalid tenements of New York City, and it is from her that our modern public health nursing and school nursing specialties arose. Wald too knew the truth of the association between the capacities necessary for a good life and the ability to conquer disease. And she knew that the work of addressing inequality in these capacities was the work of nursing.

This work is still part of the profession's DNA. Using 2001 census data on the distribution of health care professionals in England and Wales, Mary Shaw, a medical sociologist, and Danny Dorling, a human geographer, found that physicians and dentists tend to live and work in urban areas where there is greater wealth and fewer sick people, but nurses do not. Of all the health care professionals they studied, only nurses were roughly geographically distributed in proportion to the health care needs of the population. That is, medical and dental care was distributed inversely to need, but nursing care was not. Shaw and Dorling suggest that the greater the role of market forces is, the more likely that some doctors are driven by motives other than doing what is good for society. This difference can be seen, they say, "in the contrast between nurses and doctors, in terms of their choice of occupation, their salaries," and in their choice of where they live and work.

Nurses, it seems, are not as driven by market forces as other health care professionals. Indeed, in the United States, on average, registered nurses earn two-thirds less, and nurse practitioners less than half, of what physicians and surgeons earn. Perhaps nurses are driven by the profession's concern for the equal treatment of humanity. Perhaps this is why nurses tend to live and work where people most need health care, not where they will make the most money.

The profession's belief in equality and its work to bring it about are beacons in our modern times, for according to the Nobel economists Robert Shiller and Joseph E. Stiglitz, inequality defines our modern economic times and, if unaddressed, our future. Over the last thirty years, the income of the richest of society, as compared to everybody else, has shifted. The 1 percent of society that earns the most income earns, on average, more than 38 times the income of 90 percent of everybody else. This gap widens as one moves up the income gradient. The top tenth of 1 percent— the richest of the rich—earns more than 184 times the income of 90 percent of everybody else.

When it comes to wealth (that is, the value of what a person has when debts are settled), inequality is starker still. According to an Oxfam report, in 2015, the top 1 percent of the wealthiest of society had more wealth than the rest of the world put together. And in 2017, eight people—all men—had as much wealth as half of the world's population; in other words, eight men had as much wealth as roughly 3.6 billion people.

Many of these wealthiest of the wealthy have sought to do good through philanthropy. Indeed, as sociologist Linsey McGoey has chronicled, as the inequality gap has grown, the charitable sector has become one of the fastest-growing sectors of the modern economy. The consequence is, however, that large charitable organizations have replaced governments as the largest spenders on social programs and public health. This has created a situation, McGoey argues, in which billionaires wield more power on social programs and public health than governments. Billionaires, unlike governments, have no accountability to the people their philanthropic organizations serve, and when billionaires' philanthropic goals are not met, they pull their support and leave local organizations with no means to proceed. McGoey details how this creates greater inequality.

This inequality is the inequality that Shiller and Stiglitz decry. It is an inequality that is widening worldwide, and in the history of the United States, it is at its greatest ever. However, if unaddressed, it will define the future of people's capacities to lead a good life. As Wilkinson and Pickett have shown, it will lead to inequality of health outcomes. And as the top 1 percent hoard the world's wealth, the United States increasingly spends more on health care than on social services and public health, which, according to Bradley and her colleagues, will result in a future of more people with more diseases and more people who die from these diseases.

Despite the grim future inequality portends, the wealthy, who have the means to do something about it, will likely turn away. Amartya Sen, in his 1983 book *Poverty and Famines: An Essay on Entitlement and Deprivation*, documented that in four twentieth-century famines in different parts of the world that killed large numbers of poor people, there was enough food to keep everyone alive. However, in each of the four famines, this food was not shared between the wealthy and the poor. In the economic and political system of each place in which the famines occurred, the wealthy lived well fed while the poor died at their feet. Sen chronicles instances in which the wealthy brushed off starving beggars, much as I as a child saw people turning down the man begging on the streets of San Luis. In some cases, Sen notes, the wealthy saw the rotting corpses of people who had died from starvation on the streets but did nothing. The point of Sen's analysis is that the wealthy had the resources to conquer the diseases brought about by inequality, but in the case of these four famines, they did not. The wealthy did not share their wealth, not even in times when sharing would have saved lives. Rather than lose some of their food, they preferred to live in a world where corpses rotted in the street.

It seems that we cannot rely on the wealthy to address inequality in the capacities to lead a good life. They either control the purse strings of their philanthropy to the detriment of equality or ignore the effects of inequality altogether. It also seems that we cannot rely upon the health care professionals who are driven by market forces to live and work in areas of greatest need.

However, the profession of nursing has a long history of addressing the inequalities that diminish people's capacities. Nurses work among the poor, and have for well over a century. Nurses live and work in areas of greatest need. Nurses help people to center and balance their lives, even when they have disease—that is, helping them to have the freedom to choose the life they have reason to value for as long as they have life. And nurses work at all levels of nongovernmental organizations and governmental bodies to change policies that structurally reinforce inequalities. The profession of nursing promotes and restores equality in the most unequal of times and situations.

Now, many years after my summer encounter with the disabled man who begged on the street corner in San Luis, Mexico, I am still bothered by his not being whole. Maybe he had found a center and balance to his life. Maybe he had psychologically and spiritually conquered his disability. But he did not enjoy the essential capacities necessary to lead a good life, as far as I could tell. Today, as a nurse, I recognize this inequality as morally wrong, and as a nurse, I am grateful to be a member of a profession that works for equality in these essential capacities. Nursing works to make the everyday reality of people around the world match the equality of our common humanity. This is our obligation.

5

Assistance

Ruth trained at a hospital-based nursing school in 1958. She studied in the classroom in the day and cared for patients on the wards at night, catching sleep as she could. Despite being sleep deprived, nursing energized her. She liked caring for people. She felt as if she was doing good.

I came to know her some fifty years later. Even now, older and physically diminished, she walks fast, as if she is on her way to a patient who needs her. And though she is of small stature, when she slaps me on the back as she greets me, I wince from the power of her strong pitcher's arm. Her friends revel in stories about how, in her prime, she was a formidable opponent on the baseball diamond— strategically savvy but above all strong and tireless in pursuit of a win. I can only imagine her on the wards defying sleep to do what a student nurse must do: assist patients in those activities that need to be done to restore health.

At the time Ruth received her diploma and became a registered nurse, the Vietnam War raged. The nightly news brought images of injured and dying people onto the television screen in her living room. She felt overwhelmed. The sense of strength she gained from assisting the sick on the wards and in the operating room dissipated in her powerlessness to help the injured and dying on the other side of the world. Her politics were not with the war, as she once told me, but her heart was with its victims, whose suffering she could witness. They were so far away, but as a new nurse, she felt she had a duty to assist them. But how?

Most of the young American soldiers had been conscripted. If they faced injury and death out of no choice of their own, she told me, the least she could do was to choose to use the knowledge and skills she had acquired as a nurse to help them when they needed it most. She enlisted in the Air Force Nurse Corps. Straightaway, she started caring for those young men in the operating rooms of field hospitals in the war zone, and eventually, on the planes that transported them to base hospitals in Europe and the United States. Today, she speaks of her experiences only in generalities. But from what I have heard her say, I know that she assisted other flight nurses midair, and I know that she assisted young men in dying— by giving them morphine to ease their pain, by holding their hands to comfort them when that was all she had to offer, and by witnessing their last words. She did what she could to restore their health and, when there was nothing else to do, to bring as much se-renity to their deaths as possible.

The assistance Ruth gave these men is a nursing obligation. As nurses, we use our knowledge and skills to assist people in doing what needs to be done to restore or promote health or to offer peaceful deaths. As Virginia Henderson's definition of nursing instructs, this assistance is what makes nursing the profession it is; it is the profession's *sine qua non*, that without which the profession of nursing would not be nursing. At times, this assistance comes in the form of helping other health care professionals. At other times, it comes in the form of working in government or in organizations that set policies that affect people's health, managing hospitals and nursing agencies, conducting research, or educating the next gen-eration of nurses. And most often, it comes in the form of assisting others through hands-on care. In all its forms, assisting people in restoring or promoting health and in having peaceful deaths is our professional obligation.

And yet it is more than just our professional obligation. It is also our moral obligation.

This moral obligation rests in the value of our humanity. Kant, the philosopher whose idea of the categorical imperative I discussed in Chapter 2, said that this value was inestimable. Something that has a price can be replaced by something else of equal value, Kant said. But a price cannot be placed on humans, and so, the worth of human life is inestimable. If our assistance can help to restore or promote others' health, or offer them more peaceful deaths as part of respecting the inestimable value of their lives, then our professional obligation is to give it. However, our moral obligation compels us to assist others in restoring or promoting their health and in having serene deaths not because we are able to give assistance, but rather, because of the humanity of those in need of it. Another way to look at assistance as our moral obligation is to see what happens to our own humanity if we do not assist others when we can.

When we do not value others as worthy of our assistance, we place a greater value on ourselves than on them. That is, we place a greater value on our time or our energy or on our own lives than on their lives; we are unwilling to face the risks, the difficulties, or the inconveniences that may be involved in assisting them. But if it is morally legitimate to determine other people's worthiness of our assistance, other people can also determine our worthiness of their assistance, or lack thereof, should we ever need it. If we can judge others' value, others can judge ours too.

We cannot make judgments about the relative value of other humans, for when we do, we say that the worth of all humans, ourselves included, is not of inestimable value.

However, all humanity is of inestimable value—our humanity included. And because of this—because we cannot place a value on human life—we are compelled to assist others when they need assistance and we are able to give it.

Ruth knew that. On the nightly news, the newly minted registered nurse saw the young men who needed the assistance she could give. She could not sit idly by. As a young woman with few family obligations, she had the freedom to go. Unless she went, she told me, she knew she would not feel right about herself.

That is part of what it means to have a moral obligation to assist— what it means for the kind of person, not just the kind of nurse, we

are: We have chosen a profession that is defined by the obligation
to assist others. If, as nurses, we do not assist people when we can,
we devalue ourselves on two levels. First, we devalue ourselves as
nurses; we would not be faithful to what it means to be a nurse.
Second, we devalue ourselves as humans, for we would be placing
ourselves in a position of having others judge our relative value,
as we judged theirs by not assisting when we could. If, as nurses,
we abandon our obligation to assist others, we become something
other than nurses and something other than fully human, something other than a person of inestimable value, something our
nursing selves and our fully human selves could not respect. To
be nurses, we have to respect our professional obligations. In this
sense of respect, we have to recognize our professional obligations
as our personal obligations. Moreover, to respect our fully human
selves, our selves of inestimable value, we would have to choose to
act toward others as we would want them to act toward us: if we
needed assistance and someone could offer it, we would want them
to do so. And so, to respect ourselves as both nurses and humans,
we must offer the assistance of our nursing knowledge and skills to
others when they need it and we can provide it.

Thus, who we are as nurses and who we are as people are indeed
bound up together, for our professional and our moral obligation
to assist others are one and the same. In this way, the profession of
nursing assists us, as nurses, in being moral people.

Moral people, says Martha Nussbaum, are open to others and to
their plight. Fulfilling our professional obligation to assist others
opens us up to them and to their plight. We cannot be closed off to
people who need the assistance we can give. You know what this
is like in everyday life. You see the little girl riding her bicycle far
ahead of her parents. Thrilled with her newfound freedom, she
pedals faster than her balancing abilities can correct for the bump
she rides over. She tumbles and falls right in front of you. She cries.
Her parents start running toward her, but you are standing right
there. As a nurse, you go to her and, without batting an eye, you

assess her. Any bleeding? Any bones that look out of place? And so forth. In that moment of following your professional obligation you open yourself to the girl in the moment of her accident and to her parents in the moment of their helplessness. You open yourself to the point of doing what you could do to assist them, and by doing so, you fulfill your professional *and* your moral obligation.

Being open to the plight of others so that you assist them affirms the inestimable value of all humanity. It also affirms that you are worthy of being assisted by those who can do so when you need it.

Ruth could not see the injured and dying people in Vietnam on the nightly news without opening herself up to them and their plight—to their pain and suffering. When she did, she opened herself up to their humanity and was moved to the point of assisting them. She lived her professional and her personal life in accordance with the moral belief that their humanity was worthy of her assistance. Their humanity was worthy of her humanity. Their humanity and her humanity were the same.

But being open to others and to their plight also opens us up to the world that is beyond our control. This is part and parcel of being a moral person, for as Nussbaum says, the moral life is based on a willingness to being exposed. Ruth was also open in the sense that she trusted—that is, she placed herself in the hands of—the world that was beyond her control. She knew she was going into an uncertain situation in uncertain times. She knew her own life would be exposed; after all, she was going into a war zone. But she deemed her moral obligation to assist was greater than that to which she would be exposed. And she trusted that, whatever might happen to her, everything would be all right, for whatever might happen to her, she was in the right.

On a daily basis, we too expose ourselves to the uncertainties of the world when we seek to fulfill our obligation to assist others. We expose ourselves to the possibility of rejection: some people may not accept our assistance. We expose ourselves to the possibility of being used: some people may only want our assistance for their own gain, without concerning themselves to assist others when they can. We expose ourselves to the possibility of being shattered: sometimes our assistance may not be enough, and people's health might not be restored or promoted. Or sometimes, despite all that we do, some people's deaths may not be as peaceful as possible. We also expose ourselves to physical danger: we know, as nurses, that we can be exposed to life-threatening communicable diseases, and we seek to minimize this danger by using personal protective equipment and by following universal precautions. Yet despite all the equipment and all the precautions, the world remains an uncertain place. Much of what goes on is beyond our control, and when we assist others, we open ourselves up to that uncertainty.

However, not to assist others as a way of avoiding the world's uncertainties would be to create a person most of us would not want to be. It would be to create a person who would not assist out of fear of experiencing uncertainty, even though should we need assistance, we would want others to open themselves up to the uncertainty involved in assisting us. On the other hand, to follow the obligation to assist, and thus to be at risk of experiencing the world's uncertainties, is to choose to live in community with other people and to be the kind of person who assists others in their time of need. Let me illustrate with an example.

A teenage girl with mental illness was held in the custody of the state, but because she was suicidal, she needed the care that could only be provided in a specialized psychiatric hospital. However, no such hospital had appropriate space for her. The family court judge overseeing her situation remarked that he felt "ashamed and embarrassed" that the girl could not get the care she needed. The judge went on to say that the state's inability to provide proper care was a failure of its obligation toward the girl. A measure of a society, the judge suggested, is how that society assists people in need. But the judge remarked further: the failure to assist this suicidal teenage girl is "a disgrace to any country with pretensions to civilization . . . and, dare one say it, basic human decency." The measure of a society, the judge rightly notes, is bound up in the notion of human decency. I suggest that the measure of a society is society's estimation of the value of humanity. A good society—or to use his language, a society based on "basic human decency"—forms when people who have the ability to assist others in need do so, because that society believes that all human life is inestimable.

To close ourselves off to others out of fear of the risks to which we might expose ourselves is to close off the possibility of a better world. A group of people living together but not assisting each other would be something we would not call a good society. It more likely would be a dystopia in which, eventually, every person would suffer.

Even before nursing was a profession, there has never been a society without people who have filled the nursing role, and, I aver, there can never be a society without nurses. Nurses assist others in getting well, in staying well, in having babies, and in having the kind of deaths that honor humanity—assistance that is necessary for a society to be good.

When in the 1990s my wife went back to visit her childhood home in Botswana, she witnessed the cataclysmic changes the human immunodeficiency virus (HIV) epidemic had wrought—so many sickened, so many dead, so many young children orphaned; pain and suffering at every turn. It was a devastating disease that swept through the country—and through many other countries throughout the world, including the United States, which has had more acquired immune deficiency syndrome (AIDS)-related deaths per capita than any other country in the Global North.

On one trip when I went with her, we visited my wife's friend, Mpho, who was the chief nurse at an infirmary that served young adults. Mpho leapt with excitement when she saw my wife, but she looked tired, even though it was the beginning of the workday. My wife asked her if everything was all right. Mpho replied with a sigh that she had sat with a nineteen-year-old man the night before as he died. But this was her job. Besides, she had caught a few winks of sleep here and there. She was good to go, she told us. We followed her and chatted about the epidemic as she walked around the infirmary filling up large jars with condoms and straightening the "Free – Take" signs on them. She also told us about the partnership that was forming between a large American academic institution and the Botswana government to study the virus. This partnership, the Botswana Harvard AIDS Institute Partnership, is today one of Africa's leading scientific institutions. She worked with the scientists as they conducted some of their studies on the people who were in her infirmary.

After her busy work, she suggested we go outside and sit in the warm sun while we had tea. With the ambient sound of doves' cooing, we sat at a picnic table and drank strong tea heavily sweetened and slightly diluted with warm milk. After sitting in silence for a bit, Mpho told us of the agony the young man had been in the night before, not just physical agony, which she tried to palliate with pain medications, but emotional agony. She held his hand and was for him in that moment of his dying his mother, his aunt, his granny. She was for him what he needed her to be as he lay dying. She felt shattered by it all—by his death, by the manner of his death, by the deaths of so many thousands like him, by the virus's devastation of an entire generation of her country's youth, and not just her country but so many in Africa and in other continents around the world. She wept. After we finished our tea, she and my wife embraced as old and good friends. Then she brushed her clothes with her hands and said, "I have to get to back to work." Off she went into the infirmary to do what she could to restore and promote health and bring as much dignity to dying as she could in the new era of HIV. Her openness to the people who needed her assistance, the young people in her infirmary and the scientists from the partnership that was working to find treatments, struck me then, and strikes me now, as the essence of nursing's professional obligation. She did not run away from her professional obligation out of fear of being shattered physically or emotionally, but rather, she embraced it. In so doing, she embraced the inestimable value of human life, all human life—the lives of her patients, her fellow Batswana, and her own. Her professional obligation became something else: it became a way for her, a moral way of life. Her professional obligation became what she had to do to be a good person.

Almost twenty years after that day, on another visit, my wife and I sat with Mpho and her husband at a restaurant in Botswana's bustling capital city, Gaborone. Located in a new, large outdoor shopping mall, the restaurant's décor was chic and its menu Italian. Young people were everywhere, shopping and working in the mall's stores and ordering and serving food at the restaurant's tables. The difference between the 1990s and the 2010s could not have been starker. The four of us talked about it. I asked Mpho how she pushed through the hopelessness of the 1990s. She corrected me. She never felt hopeless. As a nurse, she always had something to do. She assisted the young adults who were her patients at the university infirmary. She assisted their families. She assisted the scientists. She was part of the government's working group that developed a coordinated countrywide public health response to the virus. Even now—of retirement age; her husband has, in fact, already retired— she gets up every morning and goes to work because, she says, she has something to do to contribute to the country's health.

Societies need the assistance of nurses.

After her time in the Air Force, Ruth went on to become one of the profession's leading nurse scientists. She has developed a nursing intervention that, clinical trial after clinical trial, has been proven to improve the quality of life of patients and families who are affected by life-limiting cancer. Yet today, Ruth finds herself with life-limiting cancer. Some believe that the type of cancer she has is the result of exposure to a chemical agent the United States used during the war to kill forests in Vietnam and its neighboring countries. If so, she, as with so many others during that time, opened herself up not just to being emotionally shattered by what she experienced during the war but to being physically shattered as well.

Paradoxically, she finds herself in need of the nursing assistance that she, over a lifetime of nursing, has offered to so many. As a patient, she is open to the assistance her nurses have to offer, for she knows nursing's power to heal, to bring wholeness to her life and to the lives of those who love her. She knows that when her nurses assist her, they affirm that all life, hers included, is of inestimable value. And she knows that this affirmation—an affirmation made real in everyday nursing acts of assisting the sick, the potentially sick, and the dying—is necessary to make the world a better place.

Author's Note: Ruth McCorkle (b. 1941), the Florence Schorske Wald Professor of Nursing Emerita at Yale University, passed away peacefully at home with her son, John, by her side on August 17, 2019.

6

Peace

By the 1970s, vast threats to public health from communicable diseases were diminishing. Polio was virtually eliminated, and already unheard of in the countries of the Northern Hemisphere. Smallpox was nearly eradicated, with the last known case recorded in 1977 in Somalia. New threats from diseases such as human immunodeficiency virus (HIV) were as yet unknown. The greatest threat to human health—indeed, the greatest threat to life and that which sustains life—was thermonuclear war. Nuclear bombs, if launched, would not just annihilate millions of people in moments, but make vast swaths of the earth, if not the entire planet, uninhabitable. The threat of nuclear war had become a greater threat to human health than communicable diseases.

The World Health Organization (WHO) recognized this. Of course, it was well known that, at the end of World War II, nuclear bombs killed vast numbers of people at once. But it was not until several decades later that scientists recognized the danger that the fallout produced by nuclear war tests presented to people and to the land. Exposed people were dying of cancer, and the land remained radioactive, and thus, unsafe for life. In 1973, the WHO held its first discussion on the threat nuclear war posed to health. This discussion, it might be said, began the modern-day discipline of planetary health, that is, the science and practice of caring for populations in a global context and the earth upon which our lives depend. This was indeed the concern of those gathered for that 1973 WHO discussion.

Discussions continued until 1979, when the discussants asked the WHO director-general to prepare a report on what health workers could do to address the perils that lay behind nuclear war. In 1981, seven years after discussions began, the Thirty-Fourth World Health Assembly passed resolution 34.38 to establish an international committee to write a report on how health workers can strengthen "peace, détente and disarmament and prevent thermonuclear conflict." Despite some acrimony in discussion that centered around political divides, the resolution, which affirmed that health and peace are inextricably connected, passed.

Peace is inextricably connected to health. Peace is necessary for health.

In 2016, a particular photographic image that distils the impact of war went viral on social media and in the press around the world. The photograph, taken by Mahmoud Raslan, is of a five-year-old boy who, moments before the photo was taken, had been pulled from the rubble of his bombed-out home in Aleppo, Syria. He wears shorts and a tee shirt with a cartoon figure on it. His hands are in his lap. Dried blood covers half his face. His thick black hair, styled in a bowl cut, is covered in cement dust. Staring straight ahead and seemingly unaware of the horror that had just befallen him, he sits upright on an orange ambulance seat with his hands in his lap. His face looks almost like he is ready to cry; his lips pucker. He sits alone, in no parent's lap, with no one to comfort him—containing his pain and fear as if he were a man. Yet his childhood can be seen in his little, bare feet—his tiny toes, the toes that any parent would kiss and play with, surely to his giggling delight.

What is not seen in the image most popularly reproduced, but can be found in another photograph that Raslan took with a wider angle, is a girl sitting in the seat next to the little boy. She appears to be a few years older, and she, like the boy, is dressed in summer clothes. Hers is a pink outfit with frilly sleeves. She wears a headband, which surely once held her hair in place, but now, her hair is strewn across her blood-smattered face. Like the little boy, she is barefoot. She casts her eyes downward.

The five years of fighting in Syria before this photograph was taken devastated human health. The death toll at the time of the photograph was estimated at 470,000 people, and at least 1.88 million people had sustained injury. In many parts of the country, the infrastructure for providing health care had been bombed out. The Syrian war is in no way unique. Since World War II, civilian casualties of war have only increased.

The Watson Institute for International and Public Affairs at Brown University has estimated that, in the Iraq and Afghanistan wars of the 2000s, 370,000 people died due to direct violence, but the effects of war—malnutrition, the collapse of infrastructure, and environmental degradation—had killed at least that many people. In addition, as of mid-2014, the US Department of Veterans Affairs registered almost one million disability claims related to these wars. The United Nations High Commissioner for Refugees estimated that, during 2014 and 2015 alone, 114.8 million people—about a third of the population of the United States or almost double the population of the United Kingdom—had been forcibly displaced worldwide because of violence or war.

War did not kill that little boy and girl in the ambulance in Raslan's photographs, though it most likely killed people they knew and loved. Nor, it appears from the photographs, had war maimed them. But it is clear that war had taken their innocence.

Over the last several decades, violence and war have killed, maimed, and made homeless millions and millions of people. And the threat of violence and war continues to endanger human health and that upon which human health depends. If the conditions necessary for health are incomplete without peace, then indeed, as World Health Assembly resolution 34.38 affirmed, peace is fundamental to health.

In Chapter 3, I argued that the profession of nursing has a contract with society. According to that contract, nursing promotes the health of others and the health of that upon which human health depends. If peace is necessary for human health, then nursing's contract with society is to work to promote peace.

In the seventeenth century, a pair of English philosophers, Thomas Hobbes and John Locke (whose ideas about equality I discussed in Chapter 2), gave the idea of the social contract its first full exposition and defense, perhaps in response to the English Civil War. What distinguishes Hobbes and Locke from other philosophers who have talked about the social contract, according to the contemporary essayist Elaine Scarry, is that Hobbes and Locke viewed the social contract as a "covenant for peace." Specifically, Scarry says, according to both Hobbes and Locke, the social contract is an injunction against injuring other humans. And for both Hobbes and Locke, an act that inflicts injury dissolves the social contract.

Locke's exposition of the idea of the social contract takes on special importance for health care professionals, for, as Scarry points out, Locke was first a physician and then a philosopher. As a physician, Locke was interested in the human body, particularly how people experienced pain. Scarry writes that Locke "was sensitive to other people's pain and was able to describe it with unusual vividness and precision." Indeed, for Locke, the social contract's purpose was to prevent the pain that came from bodily injury, especially bodily injury inflicted by war.

Think about how the social contract prevents bodily injury through an everyday example: an intersection of roads. We obey traffic lights at an intersection so that we do not hit an oncoming vehicle and cause bodily injury to ourselves or others. There is a temptation, when one is in a hurry, to race through an intersection when the caution light has come on. When I have done it and I am safely on the other side, I have experienced a wide-eyed fear at what I have just done. The only explanation I could give myself is that I had lost all sanity, for it is insane to risk harming others by racing through an intersection. Our behavior at an intersection—to obey the traffic lights—is an example of an agreement among members of society to behave in such a way as to prevent bodily injury. Scarry puts it this way: "The social contract prohibits us from trespassing across the boundaries of another person's body." But it is our own bodies too that we seek to protect. Part of the sobering experience after I have unwisely raced through an intersection is the thought that I could have killed myself—in addition to others. The social contract is for mutual security.

This notion that the social contract is for mutual security is Hobbes's notion. According to Hobbes, the social contract is to prevent injuries, ours and those of others, that are brought about by what he called the "miserable condition of war." The same fear of injury and death that causes us to heed the rules of the intersection, except in moments of insanity, also prevents us from warring with each other, except in moments of insanity. This fear has a positive side: the inclination toward peace. We seek peace so that we will not injure and kill each other. This, for Hobbes, is the social contract: the promotion of peace for the well-being of all. In many ways, obeying the social contract of the intersection illustrates, I think, our inclination for peace. Who wants to sustain bodily injury or death for the sake of racing through an intersection? And who wants to inflict bodily injury and death because of war? "The social contract," Scarry says, "is a contract for peace."

Nursing has a long tradition of working in conflict zones, from Florence Nightingale and Clara Barton in the nineteenth century to nurses working with international relief and medical aid agencies of today. This work addresses immediate health care needs, and it builds mutual understanding, both of which help to promote peace. It is also done out of respect for our common humanity, for these nurses deem the value of the lives of those affected by war to be of the same inestimable value as their own. However, there is a way that nurses, regardless of where they work or the circumstances they find themselves in, promote peace just by doing the work of nursing. That way is through the social contract itself, and the special features of the social contract that are part of nursing's agreement with society.

According to Hobbes, among the emotions that incline us toward peace are the desire for what we need for "commodious living" and the hope of having the means to obtain these things.

First, our work as nurses is to promote "commodious living." What patient presents to us in the clinic or the hospital who does not wish for us to improve his or her life by promoting or restoring his or her health? This is why he or she is in our care. Even the patient who presents to us as suicidal presents to us to restore him or her to a nonsuicidal state of health. Our patients want us to promote or restore their health so that they may go about living their lives. They come to us because they have a desire for "commodious living," and our work is to promote or restore their health so that "commodious living" is possible for them.

Hobbes's phrase, "commodious living," may strike our twenty-first-century ears as old and odd, but it is a wonderful phrase. "Commodious" means large, even roomy. War restricts our lives. It steals from us; it steals life and limb and, as with that boy and girl in the ambulance in Aleppo, Syria, innocence. Life in war becomes small. But life becomes large when we live peaceably with each other. Vistas of possibilities for life open up, possibilities that could not exist without peace. In war, we only live to survive, but in peace, we live beyond survival. In peace, we live looking out at life as if we are looking out at a verdant landscape. The possibilities of the good life stretch as far as the eye can see. When some of the human community live in war while others live in peace, we do not share equally in these possibilities.

The purpose for restoring and promoting health is not so that we can live in a fractured state of war in which life, if possible at all, is small. It is, rather, so that we can live large lives, full lives, healthy lives, lives of equal possibilities for leading the kind of life we have reason to value. If nursing is to promote and restore health—that is, if nursing is to work for equality in Nussbaum's capacities that are necessary for the life we have reason to value—it must also promote peace, for it is only in a state of peace that people can lead such lives.

Second, in the simplest of terms, our work as nurses gives our patients hope. When under our care, our patients need not fear a painful death, even while they are dying. When they need their health restored, we work with them so that they can regain their health. And when they need their health promoted, we help them keep their health. In all instances, nursing works with people to lead good lives, not lives riddled with fear but lives abundant with hope, hope for a future of health, even until death.

Nurses foster commodious living and give hope through their everyday work of restoring and promoting health and offering a serene death, and insofar as everyday nursing does this, it promotes peace. But there are, to my mind, two radical ways nursing promotes peace, ways that are embedded in the nature of the profession itself.

People often form social contracts within boundaries—mostly countries, but also within other alliances—and the benefits of these contracts do not extend to individuals outside these boundaries. This is not nursing's social contract. Nursing's social contract extends to all humanity, as I argued in Chapter 2. A nurse who encounters an injured person who is not his or her kith or kin cannot turn a blind eye. A nurse, to be a nurse, must care for any person who needs his or her assistance. Likewise, nursing as a profession cannot work on behalf of only certain groups. Inasmuch as nursing's work is to promote the conditions necessary for health, of which peace is one, and inasmuch as nursing cannot do so only for this or that people group, nursing must promote peace for all people, regardless of who they are or where they live. The profession of nursing, in its radically equal treatment of all people, breaks down boundaries. Nursing thus calls people to a social contract that is unbounded.

Nursing, by being the profession that it is, proclaims that, even during the anarchy of war in which the conditions necessary for health, and the conditions necessary for people to live the lives they have reason to value, do not exist, we still are one human community. Even during war, we share a common humanity. By proclaiming that nursing cares for all people, regardless of nationality, tribe, religion, sex, or gender, the profession of nursing extends to all people what Scarry calls "the equality of aliveness." Whereas war destroys lives across boundaries, nursing promotes aliveness without regard to boundaries. Nursing promotes peace by breaking down the divisions that serve as the basis for war. Nursing, in its everyday acts of caring equally for all people, makes it possible for all people to experience aliveness equally. This is the first radical way nursing as a profession promotes peace.

The second radical way is that the everyday acts of nursing are the opposite of the acts of war. Nursing mends and binds wounds. Nursing allays fears, enlarges life, and gives hope. War kills and destroys. Nursing heals. War instills fear, makes life small, and leads to despair. As the opposite of war, nursing calls people everywhere "to seek peace, and follow it," to use Hobbes's phrase. Nursing sends patients home from the hospital, the clinic, the school—the place of care—with the knowledge and skills necessary for them to continue to restore or promote their health, or to have a serene death. Nursing asks patients to go on living in a state of peace, even unto death. And nursing does this for all people—equally. Nursing fundamentally is the opposite of warring.

As I write this, nationalism is at a zenith in modern times, as I have said in the Preface and in Chapter 1. People embrace divisions, even divisions by race, ethnicity, sex and gender, and religion. Some people have based the enforcement of laws on these divisions. Moreover, language in the public square is perhaps the most bellicose I have heard in my lifetime. Nursing is poised in these times—as in all times—to proclaim the equality of all human life. Nursing is poised to proclaim the necessity of peace for health—and the good life, the life that one has reason to value. The word "peace" does not appear in the American Nurses Association's code of ethics. Yet peace and health are more than mere intellectual cousins. They are inextricably linked. To promote health, nursing must promote peace. It is our profession's obligation.

I wish I could tell you of nurses who stopped a war through their acts of caring for its victims, although I know that the work of nurses and other health care professionals has limited the effects of war. Surely there are stories of nurses who have given their lives for the purpose of peace. We would only have to go to members of the International Conferences of the Red Cross and Red Crescent—and to my colleague Ruth, who is dying of a cancer she contracted by caring for the wounded of war—to find such stories. I also wish I could tell you of people who have laid down their arms because the acts of nurses convinced them that their health and their loved ones' health, which can only be achieved through peace, are far more important than the causes of the wars they wage. What I can tell you, however, is that I have seen people affected by war. I have seen bodies maimed by armed conflict, and I have seen the faces of veterans tormented by the images of battle. But one image that will stay with me forever is of a father and a son whose lives were forever changed by war.

In the summer of 2016, I was in the Middle East working with colleagues to train cancer-care clinicians in palliative care. Every morning, I rounded with my colleagues on the palliative care unit, a unit I had been a long-term team member of seven years earlier. When I was previously there, the Syrian civil war had not yet started; in fact, it began just after I left. But by 2016, millions of Syrians were in neighboring Middle Eastern countries seeking refuge. Of course, they brought with them their maladies and need for health care. One man on the ward we visited every morning that summer of 2016 was Syrian. He was dying of cancer. It was a rare cancer that the pathologists could not pinpoint, "a cancer of unknown origin," as pathologists say. Oncologists cannot target the treatment of such cancers with precision, because treatments are based on the origin of the cancer. In this case, treatment had not slowed the growth of this man's cancer, and so, he was on the palliative care unit to die. The team wanted to enable him to die at home with home-based nursing care, surrounded by his loved ones. However, it quickly became apparent that he had no home to go to, and except for the twelve-year-old boy who was faithfully and lovingly at his side all the time, he had no one else to care for him. The father wore the effects of war on his face, a face that looked tortured. He was homeless, and he only had his young son, whom he was about to leave alone in the world.

That boy, a mere child, told us every morning how his father fared overnight. He told us when he could not rouse him, when his breathing was labored, when he was incontinent, and when his hands were cold. The boy knew his father was soon to die. The morning of the day his father died, that boy looked at the palliative care team and asked how many more hours his father had to live. In my years of nursing and witnessing people's deaths, I have never had a boy that age ask me that question. That boy had wisdom and concern that comes from years of maturity, maturity I am not sure I myself possess even now. War had stolen his innocence, just as it had stolen the innocence of that boy and girl in the ambulance in Raslan's photograph. It had also stolen his siblings and his mother. And now he was losing his father to the ravages of disease. My memory of the boy's face when he asked us how many hours his father had to live is indescribably painful. I see it again in the faces of the boy and girl sitting in the ambulance. The boy in my hospital could have known them. They could have played together. Their parents could have been friends. I do not know exactly which part of Syria the twelve-year-old boy and his dying father had traveled from. But I know that, certainly, the young children in the ambulance and the boy in the hospital room knew, in the deepest recesses of their souls, the injuries of war.

My nursing colleagues cared for that boy's father—and yes, for the boy too. I know they gave his father as peaceful a death as possible in those circumstances. I know that the long-devised plan of how to care for the boy after his father's passing was put into place by a robust social services team. However, no nurse can see that boy's face—that boy who, though not killed by war, was yet a victim of war—and say that working for peace falls outside the domain of nursing. We cannot promote health without promoting peace. The profession of nursing had a contract with that boy—and with his father. It was a contract to heal the injuries of war, even as the father lay dying. It was a contract based on the knowledge that peace is necessary for us and for our sons and daughters—and their sons and daughters, for the whole of the human community—to have health, indeed, to be able to live lives we all have reason to value. For this reason, promoting peace is an obligation of the profession of nursing.

7

Safety

I have never been as aware of our vulnerability as human beings as when my son was born. As soon as he was pulled into the air and gasped his first breath, I realized that all he could do was follow his biologic cues as his programmed cells worked together. He was circulation and respiration, intake and output. How stunning were his instincts to root for the breast and to suck. In the most profound sense, he could do nothing for himself in the world into which he had just been born. As we know, babies left alone die, and die quickly. They need our safety.

I remember the moment I knew that I would lay down my life to keep him safe. Just after he had been born, a nurse in the delivery room had taken him over to clean and weigh him under the heat lamp. I admit, I was dazed. I needed her direction. He was screaming louder than I imagined he could. His screams frightened me. In my frightened and dazed state, that nurse pushed me toward him. With her push, I followed my own instinct. I reached my index finger out to his little hand. He clenched hold of it. I have heard that newborns can hold their own weight by grabbing onto something with both fists. I do not know if this is true, but I do know that, in that moment, it seemed as if he held onto me with the force of someone who felt unsafe, and in that moment, I knew that nothing could separate me from my obligation to keep him safe. Holding him, loving him, nurturing him, and protecting him—I understood that this is what I had to do. I had an obligation to keep him safe.

He was, perhaps, at his most vulnerable at birth. Over the years, I have watched him grow up into a young man with fewer dependencies on me as a parent. But I still see his vulnerabilities. He is vulnerable to harm from accidents, disease and disorder, and natural disasters. He is vulnerable to the effects of others' actions and, of course, his own choices. And he is vulnerable to a broken heart. When I mention these vulnerabilities to him, now that he is an adult, he points out, rather deftly, that I face them too.

To be human is to be vulnerable.

To be a living thing is to be vulnerable.

We had an old copper beech tree in our yard. The official arborist where we live certified it as one of the oldest copper beeches in the area. We cared for it lovingly. The arborist told us so. We watered it during seasons of drought. We put mulch over its bare roots. We fed it the prescribed nutrients. We did everything within our power to keep this old tree alive. But we noticed that it started to look sickly. One year, its leaves came in smaller than before. It developed weeping wounds on its trunk. Some of its smaller boughs began to die. Worms started to bore into its bark. The arborist noticed it too. He diagnosed our several-hundred-year-old copper beech with a fungus. This fungus had been traveling up the eastern seaboard of the United States, felling trees on its way. We asked the arborist what to do to save our tree. He administered antifungals to its trunk. He aerated, and put minerals near, its roots. He did this for several years. But one year, when nature was waking up after the long night of a cold winter, the tree did not produce a leaf—not one leaf. It had succumbed to the fungus, which was more powerful than the available treatments. We had tried to keep it safe, but we failed. Age, the changing climate, and an opportunistic disease were stronger forces than our arbor care. The tree was gone. It was no longer vulnerable.

This is what it means to be invulnerable: not to be alive. Not to be alive, as the poet Wislawa Szymborska illustrates in his 1998 poem "Conversation with a Stone," is to lack the condition of vulnerability. We could break a stone into pieces and grind those pieces into sand, and still this sand would be the same stuff of stone, which lacks "the muscles to laugh" and has "empty" insides. Not to be alive, Szymborska's poem suggests, is to be invulnerable to that which threatens life.

Invulnerable things do not need safety in the same way vulnerable things do.

In 2015, an image gripped the world: the image of a three-year-old boy, the son of a refugee family fleeing danger at home who washed up lifeless on the sands of a Turkish beach. We felt pain at seeing the little boy lying face down and alone—dead. If he was going to die, which he should not have to do at such a tender age, should he not have died cradled in his mother's loving arms? How could I as a father not feel the horror of his death? What if my son were to drown at sea and be washed up—alone!—on the shores of an unknown place? The unspeakable—the irreplaceable—loss! We all—the entire human community—failed to provide that little boy safety from the seas upon which he and his family had sailed trying to find safety, trying to find the conditions necessary for them to be able to lead lives they had reason to value. He, a mere child—someone's son, grandson, brother, and playmate, and someone's hope for the future—had been helpless in his short life. He needed our safety. He died without it.

Human life cannot be replaced; it cannot be compensated for. What dollar figure could I ever—would I ever—place on that little boy or on my own son? Because human life is of inestimable value, we have an obligation to provide safety to those who are at risk of succumbing to the vulnerabilities of being alive. This obligation is fundamental to the profession of nursing. You cannot be a nurse and not believe that it is your duty to provide safety.

As nurses, we care for the sick to give them safety from their vulnerabilities. We use our expert knowledge and skills to fend off their diseases. We give them time to repair and the space to heal. We know that the middle-aged person coming into our emergency department with chest pains may be having a heart attack. We move into quick action to do everything we can to clear blocked cardiac arteries and, we hope, to prevent permanent heart damage or even death. And then we provide bedside care, calm fears, and educate about lifestyle changes that can reduce future risks of heart disease. The sick come to us for safety from that which threatens their lives so they can heal and once again, with knowledge about how to keep themselves safe, face life's challenges.

The same is true of those who are potentially sick. We perform well visits to prevent diseases, and thus, provide safety from that to which people might otherwise succumb. We give vaccinations for communicable diseases that, not long ago, decimated and maimed large swaths of humanity. We screen for cancers to catch them while they are still highly treatable. And we educate on how to lead healthy lives. We provide nursing care so that those who are well can remain well. This is to provide safety.

We also care for the dying, who are vulnerable to unwanted suffering. When we provide hospice and palliative nursing care, we make it possible for people to be safe from needless suffering as they die, and we shelter their loved ones from the greater grief tumultuous deaths bring.

Providing safety for the sick, the potentially sick, and the dying is what we do as part of our everyday work as nurses. In so doing, we respect their humanity. They likewise respect our humanity, and in this mutual respect lie the bonds of the social contract, the contract upon which not just peace but also health is maintained.

Yet some people are more vulnerable than others. Their safety is at greater risk. To them we owe a greater obligation. This is why we assess people for risk of abuse, neglect, or harm. It is also why we are mandated by law to report suspicion that a child, a dependent adult, or an older person has been abused or neglected, or when we suspect that people are at risk of harming themselves or others. As a civil society, we recognize that there are members of society who, because of the conditions of their lives, are more vulnerable to threats to their humanity, and hence, need our protection more. But we owe the protection of our safety not just to the populations the law deems as more vulnerable.

We also owe the protection of our safety to people who are made more vulnerable by structural inequalities. Structural inequalities are inequalities in housing, income, education, and the criminal justice system, and inequalities that arise from being a member of an underrepresented group—a group that can be differentiated from those who hold most social and political power. Because people who experience structural inequalities are more vulnerable, we as a profession have a greater obligation to provide them safety from the vulnerabilities these inequalities pose, as I argued in Chapter 4.

This obligation is rooted in the profession's identity as a compassionate profession. But compassion is complex. It is both emotion and thought, and it lives in the interstices of human interaction. It is, as Martha Nussbaum says, "the basic social emotion," an emotion that carries with it logical implications for the way we function in society.

When we see others experiencing something we ourselves would not want to experience, we recognize a vulnerability we would not want to face ourselves. In this recognition, we feel the wrong—the moral wrongness—of someone having to experience such a thing. This is what I felt when I looked at the picture of the little boy dead on the beach. I would not want to experience losing my son the way that little boy died. Nor would I want my son to die that way. I felt the wrong of it. Compassion is feeling the wrongs of what others experience—the wrongs we would not want to experience ourselves. Compassion is a crucial aspect of the common humanity I discussed in Chapter 2.

When we feel compassion, we recognize that bad things might happen to us too. According to Nussbaum, we estimate the meaning of another's suffering by thinking about what it would mean to encounter that suffering ourselves. We see ourselves as people to whom such things might happen in the future. Nussbaum says that this is one reason compassion and fear are close to each other. We do this as mothers and fathers, brothers and sisters, partners and lovers, friends and strangers, nurses and patients. We think about what it would mean for us, or for those whom we love, to experience something bad, such as a lonely, violent death at sea, and we are afraid of it happening to us or to those whom we love. The compassion I felt for that little boy, and for his loved ones, sits very near to the terror I feel at the thought of that happening to my son. In our fearful recognition, we form the bond of our common humanity with those to whom something bad has happened, and in this bond, we respect their—and our own—humanity. We respect the fact that if what happened to them would be bad for us, it *is* bad for them. The us-them distinction falls away in our common humanity. If what happened to them would be bad for us, then it *is* bad for any human being.

In the absence of compassion, we behave as if we are above life's vulnerabilities. This leads us to "treat other people in ways that inflict . . . miseries [we] culpably fail to understand," Nussbaum says. To believe we are above life's vulnerabilities is to believe that we are invulnerable. To be invulnerable is to be inhuman, as Szymborska's poem illustrates. But through compassion, we acknowledge our common vulnerabilities: to be human, after all, is to be vulnerable. Through compassion, we enlarge our own humanity.

But compassion is more than an emotion.

Compassion is also thinking about what humans ought to have by virtue of being human. As a profession, nursing holds that all people ought to have equal access to the capacities essential for health and well-being, and as a profession, nursing takes notice of people who experience structural inequalities that impede equal access to these capacities. Nursing takes special notice when they suffer poor health outcomes because of these structural inequalities. In response, we say that no human being should experience such inequalities and the poor outcomes that result. This is a place where human rights do come into play. Every human has a right to equality in the structures of society that are necessary for health. This right is based on our common humanity: if structural inequalities are bad for one, they are bad for all. But as we saw in Chapter 3, human rights are pleas (demands, in many cases) for others to fulfill their obligations. Obligations logically come before rights. Rights come most prominently into play when we are disenfranchised from them. When we see people cut off from their rights, we have an obligation to act to enfranchise them. This is the rational aspect of compassion: thinking about what is right and what we are obligated to do when we encounter wrongs.

Therefore, compassion requires action. It would be cruel not to act once one feels the wrongs visited upon others. It would also be cruel not to act once one thinks about what is right for others who have been wronged—by structural inequalities. Compassion changes you. You cannot un-feel the wrongs once you have felt them. You cannot un-know that which you know is right. If you are bound to others who experience wrongs because you would not want to experience these wrongs yourself, and if you are led by these feelings to think about what is right for others—and thus for yourself and the entire human community—then you cannot sit by and watch these wrongs go unmitigated, those rights left unfulfilled. If you do, you are not doing right by yourself, much less by others. Rather, to do right by yourself and others, you must act to right the wrongs others experience.

More important, inaction would be the opposite of compassion. Inaction would be to think that you are not bound to others who experience bad things. Inaction would be to inflict more suffering on others by doing nothing but merely being a voyeur. In their suffering, they become our amusement. If, however, nursing is to remain a compassionate profession, as nurses, we must feel compassion when others are wronged. We must think about what is right. And we must act to provide safety, especially when people's health is made more vulnerable by structural inequalities, for these are wrongs that we ourselves would not want to experience. We cannot wish these wrongs to be universal. They violate the respect we owe our common humanity. And thus, we have an obligation to act.

All health care professions have an obligation to provide safety, but nursing has a special obligation. This special obligation goes to the heart of the profession. Nursing is not the art and science of preventing, diagnosing, and treating disease and disorder; that is medicine. Insofar as medicine does this in a way that is equal for all people, it meets its obligation to provide safety. Nursing's obligation, however, is not just to maintain health among the well and to treat the diseases of the sick. Nursing's obligation is to be a human profession that understands that the lot of the most vulnerable among us is the lot of all of us. As clergyman and antiwar activist William Sloane Coffin Jr. said of the profession, nursing "keep[s] everything together." Nursing holds together the rich and the poor, the fed and the hungry, the free and the persecuted, the sheltered and those who hide from the weapons of war. Compassion, in nursing, means holding everything together.

By holding everything together, nursing provides safety to the human community. This is the image I see in poet Emma Lazarus's depiction of Florence Nightingale as Lady Liberty: a nurse providing safety to the tempest-tossed. That little boy who lay dead on a Turkish beach, whose death was the result of the structural inequalities of war, had a right to safety. We, as a human community and especially as a profession rooted in compassion, had an obligation to keep him safe, an obligation we collectively failed to keep.

Nursing, if it is anything, is a profession that provides safety.

When, collectively as nurses, we take a stand between the most vulnerable and the most powerful—between the tired, the poor, the homeless, and the tempest-tossed, and the powerful whose policies have made them that way—we say to the powerful that they are no safer than those whom they make unsafe. When we call the powerful to even out the structural inequalities of society, we call for an enduring safety. This enduring safety is built upon nursing's vision of the equality of all humanity, for ultimate safety is found when all humans share the same level of vulnerability. Unless the powerful feel their real, human vulnerability, they make the world unsafe. Nursing calls the powerful to account for their role in the (un)safety of all humans.

This is our profession's obligation of safety: to work toward ensuring that no one person is more vulnerable than another by virtue of structural inequalities. And this obligation extends not only to the human community but also to the earth upon which the human community depends.

8

Earth

The copper beech tree that stood in our yard witnessed many a family living in our house, many a passerby on the sidewalk, and many a child playing under its shade. For years, it took in carbon dioxide these people exhaled and, in exchange, produced oxygen. It was a member of the array of living things on Earth that makes this planet our home in the vast expanse of the universe. Earth is where we live. It is where we find food, water, and shelter. It is where we came to be, and when we die, it is where our bodies will repose. Without Earth—without the intricate balance of life upon it, and the protection of the atmosphere above it—we simply would not be. But because of how we treat Earth, it is under threat. How we live on it matters for our lives and for lives yet to come. For the sustenance of human life—indeed, for life itself—we have an obligation to Earth.

Earth is in peril, and its peril is because of how we humans have lived and continue to live. In acknowledgment of humans' effect upon Earth, scientists have named this geologic age the Anthropocene. A contemporary atmospheric chemist and Nobel laureate, Paul Crutzen, first proposed the concept of the "Anthropocene" to capture what he calls "a quantitative shift in the relationship between humans and the global environment."

The origins of the Anthropocene are embedded in human history. Early humans made tools and weapons to their purposes. They could hunt, and with the manipulation of fire, they could keep dangerous animals away. As humans continued to develop, they started to clear forests and till the land. Then, as their numbers grew, they formed large-scale communities, and over millennia, civilizations rose and fell. And yet during that time, as climate scientists Will

Steffen, Jacques Grinevald, John McNeill, and Crutzen himself say, the extant geologic data suggest that humans maintained a healthy relationship with Earth. It is only with the Industrial Revolution that the human community exited this relationship, and the Anthropocene began in earnest.

Until the Industrial Revolution, energy sources were all solar in one way or another: Plants and animals, which depend upon photosynthesis, were sources of energy. So were wind and water. Wind patterns and the hydrological cycle are influenced by the sun. But the discovery and exploitation of fossil fuels—first, coal in 1748; natural gas in 1821; and then petroleum in 1859—represented a source of solar energy that was not dependent on the vagaries of photosynthesis, atmospheric circulation, and the hydrological cycle. Fossil fuels, which accumulated over hundreds of millions of years, are a dense and easily transported energy source stored deep underground. With the technology of the Industrial Revolution, these vast underground storage containers became accessible, and with mass extraction, fossil fuels became affordable.

With this abundant and dependable energy source, humans undertook new and more activities. Factories were invented to mass-produce goods. Forests were converted into grazing areas and croplands on a grand scale, and with the invention of fertilizer, which fossil fuels made possible, agriculture moved from small family-run farms to vast corporate enterprises. Water was diverted with large-scale dams that were constructed with the heavy equipment fossil fuels made possible. Fossil fuel–powered steam, internal combustion, and reactive engines extraordinarily accelerated movement across Earth's surface. Nowadays, trains, cars, jets, and rockets get us from here to there with a speed and ease unimaginable before the Anthropocene. With this use of fossil fuels came a greater atmospheric concentration of the gases they emit—the gases we have come to call greenhouse gases because, like the glass of a greenhouse, they trap heat within the atmosphere and cause the climate to warm.

Steffen, Grinevald, Crutzen, and McNeill detail the dramatic increase in such atmospheric-imprinting human activity in a now-legendary 2011 article. Between 1800 and 2000, they say, Earth's human population grew six-fold, but energy use grew forty-fold and economic production fifty-fold. During this two-hundred-year period, the greatest acceleration in human activity came after World War II. This accelerated activity's effect on the global environment is clearly discernable, Steffen, Grinevald, Crutzen, and McNeill say. They warn: If the human activities that drive the Anthropocene—such as fossil fuel use, deforestation, intensive livestock production, and use of synthetic fertilizers—"continue unabated through [the twenty-first] century, [they] may well threaten the viability of contemporary civilization and perhaps even the future existence of *Homo sapiens*." Will we escape our demise by our own hand?

This is not a hypothetical question. As I write, the United Nations' Intergovernmental Panel on Climate Change has just released a scientific report that describes the consequences of the already-warming climate, for example, more extreme weather, rising sea levels, and diminishing Arctic sea ice, among other changes. Because of the warming climate, fifty million people will be exposed to the effects of increased flooding. The availability of clean, fresh water will decrease. Food insecurity will increase from decreased crop, livestock, and aquaculture production. Because of hotter, drier weather, wildfires will devastate vast swaths of forests and scrub land, and because of warming seas, coral reefs, on which a quarter of sea life depends for health, will die. These effects of the warming climate, among others, will be felt on every inhabited continent and every ocean on Earth. The scientists who wrote the report portend a world crisis by 2040 if we do not act now.

This should concern us as nurses, in part, because of the inevitable effects on human health. In 2016, the US Global Change Research Program issued a startling report on these health effects. Rising sea levels and more intense weather events will contaminate water; they will also displace people, disrupt ways of life, and destroy livelihoods. Longer and more intense heat waves have caused, and will continue to cause, more heat-related illnesses and deaths. Hotter temperatures will increase the number and the severity of wildfires, which will worsen air quality and result in more acute and chronic heart and lung diseases, and from these diseases, more premature deaths. Hotter temperatures will also allow for disease-carrying mosquitoes to live in places they otherwise would not, to live longer, and thus, to transmit disease to more people. The same is true for other vectors of disease, such as ticks. Pathogens that thrive on heat and humidity, such as *Salmonella*, will become more active and contaminate more food products, which will lead to more food-related infections. There will be mental health effects: more distress, more behavioral health disorders—for example, from exposure to traumatic weather-related disasters—and, from increased deaths, more grief. These effects will be felt more intensely by those who experience structural inequalities, particularly those who experience poverty.

Regardless of where the poor live—in low-, middle-, or high-income countries—they disproportionately face the loss of means of living, and loss of life itself, from extreme weather events related to the warming climate. For example, the geography of Bangladesh makes it prone to flooding. A scientific report by the World Bank suggests that warming climate–related flooding will increase in Bangladesh, where the poor, because of the vulnerability of their living situations, will be most affected. They will lose their means of food production, their livelihoods, and their lives more than the rich.

In the United States, Alaska has warmed twice as fast as the global average. Arctic sea ice has melted, which has caused the sea level to rise. Permanently frozen subsoil, known as permafrost, has now thawed. Permafrost keeps the land habitable along the northwestern Alaskan coast. Less permafrost has meant less land to live on. The rising sea level and less habitable land have displaced Alaska Native communities along the northwestern coast. That is, instead of being internally displaced by war, Alaska Natives are internally displaced by the warming climate. A Brookings Institution report, *Climate-Induced Displacement of Alaska Native Communities,* describes the devastating effects of entire communities having to be relocated because of the warming climate: ancestral villages have been lost to the rising sea, traditional ways of life have been forever altered, and poverty has increased from the loss of fishing livelihoods. Even before this devastation, Alaska Natives have been among the poorest people in the United States. And it is we who have done this: through our climate-warming activities, we have increased the vulnerability of an already-vulnerable population.

Indeed, if the climate scientists are to be believed, the most vulnerable are the canaries in the climate's coal mine. Their fate will one day be the fate of all, rich and poor alike.

Florence Nightingale knew the importance of Earth to nurses' essential function: promoting and restoring health. In her 1860 *Notes on Nursing,* she put forward what we have come to call the environmental theory of nursing. Nightingale's theory is straightforward: as nurses, we are to use the environment to promote or restore a patient's health. She admonishes nurses to keep water clean and to make sure the air the patient breathes is as pure as possible. In fact, keeping the air pure is her first rule of nursing. Actually, the first rule is to keep the air the patient breathes as pure as the outside air. But the outside air is no longer pure and, according to a US government study, the drinking water available to many people in the United States, one of the most developed countries in the world, is filled with high levels of toxic chemicals. How can we nurses use the environment—how can we use pure air and clean water—to promote and restore health? In the Anthropocene, Nightingale's environmental theory necessarily invokes environmental ethics. To use the environment for healing—to use Earth for healing—it becomes a professional obligation to promote and restore Earth's health. Our ability to promote and restore our patients' health depends, ultimately, on the health of Earth.

My argument thus far has been that the warming climate affects human health. These effects fall more heavily upon the vulnerable. And because of the warming climate's effects on Earth's health, nurses' ability to restore and promote human health is diminished. As nurses, these are good enough reasons to be concerned about Earth. But we are not just nurses; we are members of the human community. I now turn to moral philosophy to argue the reason the human community as a whole should be concerned about Earth's health. That reason is, simply put: Earth has moral standing of its own.

Earth gives us the only home we have. It is not just any home, however. It is the only planet where we can live in our natural state. That is, we are dependent upon Earth for our lives. Because of this dependency, we should treat Earth with special regard. This line of reasoning is valid, but it still is focused on us as the human community, that is, on what Earth does for us.

Earth's moral standing, however, is not because we depend upon it. It is, rather, that what we do to Earth changes it in irrevocable ways, as the UN report on climate change details. Our activity forever alters Earth and may forever alter its ability to be home to all the living things that depend upon it, ourselves included. In a most profound way, our activity alters Earth's ability to do what *it* is supposed to do. Our activity alters *Earth's* natural functioning. Herein we see Earth's moral standing: Earth's inherent nature (its quiddity; its essence) is to be *the* place where the things that can only live upon it can indeed live upon it. During the Anthropocene, we, the human community, have changed Earth so drastically that the things that can only live upon Earth soon may not be able to live upon it. We are in the process of changing Earth's inherent nature.

Because we, the human community, are in the process of changing Earth's inherent nature—and thus, violating its moral standing—our actions are immoral. Earth was here before each of our lives and will exist after, we hope. Yet we have sought to take dominion over Earth, rather than living in a guest-host relationship with it. During the Anthropocene, we, the human community, have become destructive to Earth.

Is there anything in this moral argument that concerns us as nurses specifically and not just as members of the human community? That is, what are we, the community of nurses, to do to make this right? Do we have a professional obligation toward Earth? I would argue that we do.

The profession's obligation, of course, entails public health policies and position statements by professional associations that address changing behaviors that lead to the warming climate. The profession's leading association, the International Council of Nurses (ICN), has done this. The ICN gives practical recommendations on what the profession can do at the global, national, and personal levels; these recommendations are in the appendix to this book. At the heart of all these recommendations is an ethic of working together—across national boundaries and societal differences, even across beliefs about what needs to be done. Environmental ethics (that is, our obligation to Earth) is to work "together across all our diverse and unequal social worlds," as the contemporary geography and environmental systems scientist Erle C. Ellis says.

As individuals, we can do this. We *can* choose to live in ways that promote and restore Earth's health. In addition, as a part of the health care sector, we can call the health care industry to lead by example. As the scientists who wrote the UN climate change report say, there is no way to reverse or even slow the declines in Earth's health and the effects these declines have on all life, including the human community, without changing how we live and work. As nurses, we need to do our part to reduce health care waste and to implement Earth-friendly policies in our clinics and hospitals. We need to teach the next generation of nurses that the care of Earth is at the heart of the profession. As nurses, we are to promote and restore health. It is just that now, we can no longer think only of people when we say this. We must include Earth's health.

If, as Virginia Henderson said, the unique function of the nurse is to assist the individual in those activities that restore or promote health, then today, in the age of the Anthropocene, this unique function necessarily includes those activities that restore and promote Earth's health. As the world's largest profession, we can work together across our diversity, across our different social and political worlds, to do this.

In December 1968, rockets attached to the Apollo 8 spacecraft hurtled three men out of Earth's orbit. They sped through darkness and, with precise calculations and exact maneuverings, voyaged into the moon's orbit. Once there, they could see Earth rise out of the darkness of space, just as we on Earth see the sun rise out of the darkness of night. These astronauts were, in fact, the first to see—and to photograph—Earth rising. In a *New York Times* documentary, Emmanuel Vaughan-Lee interviews these men about their experience. They stumble for words. One even suggests that he could not describe what he felt when he saw Earth rising on the horizon of the galaxy's great darkness. Instead of sending an astronaut into space, he said, "they should've sent a poet." Seeing his home planet dangle in the vast expanse of space was the kind of awe-inspiring experience that only a poet could try to put into words. This awe at Earth being what it is deepens when we think about what Earth is to us. More profoundly, we are obliged to care for its health because of what Earth is in and of itself: the only home for life that can only live upon it.

Two things inspired awe in Immanuel Kant: morality and the starry heavens above. Drawing from Kant's thought, I suggest that, when from their vantage point within the starry heavens they saw Earth rising, those astronauts felt the awe of Earth having a moral status of its own. This moral status places upon us, the nursing profession, a profession of healers who can only live upon Earth, an obligation to promote its health.

9
Respect

Gordon Kamara was an ambulance nurse in Monrovia, Liberia, during the 2014 Ebola outbreak there. He picked up patients from their homes, where they lay bleeding to death. He picked up others off the city streets where they had fallen ill while out shopping. The *New York Times* video journalist Ben C. Solomon interviewed Gordon as he put a patient into his ambulance. Gordon told Solomon how he felt he had to care for these patients, despite the danger to his own health; he *had* to be an ambulance nurse during the Ebola crisis. He lamented the many lives lost to the virus, including some members of his own family. He also lamented how his work took him away from his partner and their six children. He did not go home to them at night for fear of passing the virus on to them, should he have contracted it unawares. He told Solomon that he hoped for the day when Ebola could be contained, even cured.

Now, some years after Solomon interviewed Gordon, good progress is being made on public health initiatives that contain the virus. Progress is also being made on a vaccine. But during the height of the epidemic, when Liberians feared for their lives, Gordon cared for the sick with the only means he had available. As he helped an older woman into his ambulance, he turned to Solomon's camera and said, "The first thing I do, I give them courage. I tell them, 'Don't be afraid.' They feel fear. I see it in their eyes," he said. "I am tired of seeing people getting sick." All Gordon had was his care—his taking care to give the sick courage to face the challenges that lay ahead. And this care was good.

On these front lines of the Ebola crisis, Gordon's idea of what was good was to transport the sick to where they could get the intensive care they needed and instill in them courage. Yes, his idea of what was good extended to a world in which, through the advances of science, the power of the virus would be vanquished, a world in which the virus would no longer kill. But he was not a virologist; he was a nurse. And so as a nurse, he did what he could. "Don't be afraid," he told his patients. "I will care for you."

Gordon's idea of caring for the sick was not just his idea of what was good—it was his idea of what was good for him *to do with his life*. It was his idea of a life he had reason to value. And as we can tell from his devotion, he elevated caring for the sick above all other concerns. He valued it and his life of doing it.

Gordon's caring acts show forth the moral character of nursing—that is, the primacy of the good of caring for the potentially sick, the sick, and the dying.

More profound, however, is that the profession's moral character also became Gordon's. The good of nursing became that which he valued. Philosophically, this is the same unity of professional and personal morality as I described in Chapter 5, where I discussed assistance. I can imagine that Gordon's partner and his six children argued and pleaded with him not to be an Ebola ambulance nurse. I would not have faulted him if he felt his loyalties lay with them before the Ebola-stricken people of Monrovia. But he needed to be an ambulance nurse to pursue what, for him, was of value. His plan for his life as a nurse was good—good for him and, surely, good for those for whom he cared. And because he valued his plan for his life as an Ebola ambulance nurse, it was worth doing.

If you have made nursing your life, what you do as a nurse brings good into the world. You could have chosen another profession with doing good in mind. You could have chosen to become a teacher, a charity worker, an engineer, a doctor, a virologist, a firefighter—all of whom do good through their work, immeasurably so. But you chose to be a nurse. As a nurse, your idea of what is good is bound up in what you do day in and day out. Your idea of what is good has something to do, I suspect, with the value you place on your everyday nursing activities, or else you would not be a nurse. You may have a humble job, picking up the sick off the streets of Monrovia, emptying bedpans full of what Nightingale called the "noxious effluvia" of nursing, or changing the intravenous bag of normal saline for a patient who is dehydrated. Humble though these jobs may be, these are good activities. By doing them, you do good.

Nursing activities are good in and of themselves, independent of your valuation of them. However, as well as carrying out good acts, you, as with Gordon, can consciously choose to see your nursing activities as good. If you see your nursing activities as good, then you see yourself as contributing to a better world. And if you see yourself as contributing to a better world through your work, then your plan for your life as a nurse is worth carrying out.

Self-respect, according to the philosopher John Rawls, is the confidence that your plan for your life is worth carrying out. A nurse who chooses to see his or her work as good has the confidence that it is worthy of dedicating his or her working life to. He or she has reason to live the life he or she values.

At first, this seems a tautology, an empty truth. If a nurse takes nursing as worthy of dedicating his or her life to, then of course he or she values it, for how could he or she not value that which is, by definition, good? How could he or she not value doing good?

Part of what is good about nursing activities is that they are just that: actions in the here and now. As I have argued throughout this book, ideas without actions are meaningless. A nurse's idea of what is good is not a fantasy—a mere quixotic daydream—about a utopia that will never come about. On the contrary, a nurse's idea of what is good necessarily involves everyday nursing activities, activities in the present, which are good in themselves. And so, a nurse's idea of what is good does not derive from an action-less idea, but rather, from his or her everyday good nursing activities. Gordon calmed the old woman he put into his ambulance. He gave her courage, even though he knew the likelihood that she would die from Ebola was far greater than the likelihood that she would live. Giving her courage through his care was his nursing activity, and it was good. It was not a mere idea. It was a good act.

It is thus not an empty truth to say that a self-respecting nurse is confident that his or her plan for his or her working life is worth pursuing, for he or she can rightly be confident in the good that he or she does. But when a nurse fails to value his or her activities, he or she does not see them as contributing to what is good, even though they do. If a nurse does not value his or her nursing activities, he or she does not value his or her work. He or she does not have confidence that his or her working life is worthy of doing. The nurse lacks self-respect.

As nurses, we have an obligation to have confidence in the value of what we do. If we do not, then we should not be nurses.

It is often difficult to see the value of what we do, day in and day out. We often have too many patients during our shifts to provide safe, much less high-quality, care. We sometimes get forced into overtime so our nurse managers can ensure that necessary nurse-to-patient ratios are maintained. When this happens, it affects other parts of our lives. It makes us doubt the value of our life plan to be a nurse.

I often was asked to stay late in the clinic. Because my wife frequently travels for work, I had contingency plans for picking up my son from the school's aftercare program when this happened. However, one winter night, all of my "plan Bs" fell through. It was every parent's nightmare. I could see my son standing in the dark, cold winter night, alone on the steps of the school, abandoned by his overworked and grouchy father. I could see myself racing to the school, screeching my car's tires as I turned the corner, only to see his forlorn face and the scowl of the afterschool teacher, whom I had also made stay. That night—that dark, cold winter night—when I needed to leave the clinic on time and it seemed as if I would not make it to my son's school in time to get him, it was hard for me to believe in the value of what I did. I admit: I wanted to quit.

Gordon, certainly, must have had his moments of wondering whether his plan for his life as a nurse was worthy of doing. Solomon films Gordon in his temporary housing, the housing he chose to stay in rather than expose his family to the virus should he have caught it. He sits on his bed and shows Solomon pictures of his partner and their children. He cries and says that he can only say goodnight to them by saying goodnight to their photos. He tenderly kisses the photos and then pins them back onto the headboard of his makeshift bed. How could he not have had doubts? His own life and the well-being of his family were at stake. There are many nurses around the world who risk much for the sake of pursuing their plans to be nurses. But they take these risks because they have confidence in the value of their life's work. And because they do, they have self-respect.

Self-respect is confidence in what one does with one's life, even if there are costs and perils along the way. This confidence makes us better at what we do, for when we have confidence in what we do—confidence in what we have been educated to do and in what we are good at doing—our ability to do it grows. A novice nurse, for instance, needs to be trained and needs to practice what he or she has been trained to do. If the nurse has confidence in what he or she has been trained to do, he or she will practice it even more. Over time, the nurse's confidence will grow, and as it does, his or her abilities will grow too. Eventually, he or she will not have to think about the steps involved in the tasks in which he or she has been trained; he or she will have practiced them so much. His or her practice will become second nature, and he or she will have an intuitive grasp of what he or she does. The nurse will come to the place in his or her skill at which he or she will not have to think much about what he or she is doing. The nurse will operate from a deep confidence in what he or she does, and because of this confidence, his or her performance will become fluid, flexible, and proficient; and when his or her performance is thus, he or she is an expert. Our confidence in the value of what we do allows us to become better and better at it, until we become experts.

In this way, self-respect is a social good, Rawls says, for it enables us to become better at what we do, and this betterment in itself is good. Self-respect brings the good of becoming expert at what we do. Self-respect begets good. This is why we have an obligation to respect ourselves: because we have an obligation to do good.

At the same time that we have an obligation to self-respect, the profession has an obligation to create the conditions necessary for self-respect. Creating these conditions is a sign that the profession values what we, everyday nurses, do; that is, creating these conditions is the profession's way of having confidence in us nurses.

When we do not feel valued by our profession, it is difficult for us to enjoy our work. As a result, we may become slack. Our skills may wane, and when they do, we may rightly lose confidence. When we lose confidence, we no longer see how our activities contribute to that which is good. And then it is easy for us not to see what we do as nurses as worthy of our time and energy. We feel disillusioned. Disillusionment is the loss of faith in what we do; it is the loss of faith in our profession. When we are disillusioned, we do not have confidence in our plans for our lives as nurses. We devalue our lives as nurses, and then we lose self-respect.

But when we have self-respect, we see each other's contribution to the good, through our nursing activities, as valuable. And this value is equal; through our nursing activities, we contribute equally to that which is good. You may not be on the front lines of a public health crisis, but you do good as a nurse. The good that Gordon did is equal to the good of the cardiac nurse, the surgical nurse, the maternal-newborn nurse, the school nurse, the hospice nurse. When we have confidence in the good that we do ourselves, we see the good that each of us does. And because we see that we all do good, we see the difficulties each of us faces in trying to do good. We see others' points of view.

That is, we see others' points of view as worthy of regard. When I was asked to stay late at the clinic, I explained to my manager why I could not. All my "plan Bs" had fallen through. The truth is, being a good father figures into my idea of what I value just as much as my being a good nurse. I did not then—nor do I now—see these two aspects of my life as competing. In fact, I think being a good nurse contributes to my being a good father, and vice versa. But there were times, it seemed to me, that my manager thought they were competing. Or rather, there were times when I thought that she did not see my need to pick up my son before aftercare closed as part of my idea of what I valued. I wondered whether she could see my point of view, that is, if she could understand my reason for requesting not to stay late. If she could not understand my reason, how could I value the work that I did under her management?

Respecting another person's reasons for what he or she values is essential, for it communicates—in deed, not just in idea—the belief that another person's reasons are equal to our own. It is the acknowledgment of the mutuality of our situation. It is to take on each other's problems, to be one human community. To respect another person's reasons for what he or she values is to respect our common humanity. It is to see, reflexively, that that which others value is of value to us as well.

The nurse manager had good reasons for requiring someone to stay after his or her shift was done. I too had a good reason for saying that I could not. I knew my manager would be affected by my not staying late, and I owed her my reason. She too had to be willing to give me her reason for her request, as her request directly affected me—*and my son.* This kind of valuing one another—this willingness to see a situation from another's point of view and to give reasons for our actions when they affect others—is what Rawls calls mutual respect.

By now, you probably have guessed how my predicament resolved. Another nurse, a woman at a different life stage (her children were away in college), said, "Go get your son, Mark. I'll stay." She saw the situation from my point of view. She respected my reason for not being able to stay late, and she made it possible for me to do that which I valued: to be a good nurse *and* a good father. She also respected the nurse manager's reason for needing someone to stay late: The nurse who was supposed to come on shift after us had called out sick. A replacement nurse was needed so that patients could be safely cared for. *It was good for one of us to stay late* until a replacement nurse could be called in; I valued this. The nurse manager needed to make sure the patients in her ward received good nursing care. If you have ever been a patient, you know that the nurse manager's reason was, indeed, good. The respect that my colleague showed me and our nurse manager, the respect that my nurse manager showed me for valuing my reason for not being able to stay late, and the respect we showed our patients for heeding the right nurse-patient staffing ratio was, at its essence, mutual respect. Mutual respect, Rawls says, is simply treating others fairly.

To treat each other fairly is to form a microcosm of a good society. It is to be a community of equals, even though some of us may be on a lower pay grade than others. It is to be a community in which we share problems and seek solutions to them equally. It is to be a community in which we respect ourselves and each other.

As a good society, the profession of nursing could show others what such a society is, a society in which all humans respect each other. Much of what is going on with the profession—with low retention and high job dissatisfaction rates—is that, in many ways, workplaces (and by extension the profession) do not respect nurses equally. Disillusionment, the loss of faith in what we do, results from this inequality of respect, as do dissatisfaction and discontentment. Inequality, as I argue in Chapter 4, disrespects our common humanity.

Our work and our plans for our lives can take different forms. There is not just one way for nurses to make good contributions to the profession and to society. For instance, in academic nursing, the science and the art of nursing contribute equally to the profession and to society. Nurses at the bedside, chief nursing officers and nurse managers, nurses in policy and advocacy—all contribute equally to the good of the profession and society. Because we all, in our various roles, contribute equally to what is good, we are obligated to respect each other. And when we who form the profession of nursing respect each other, nursing then is a fair profession.

In mutual respect we find confidence in the good that we collectively do with our working lives as nurses. Mutual respect and self-respect cannot be untangled. To have confidence in the good of nursing, we first must have confidence in the good that we do as nurses. It is our obligation to respect the goodness of our nursing activities, the activities of caring for the potentially sick, the sick, and the dying. They are, after all, good deeds.

PART III

NURSING BEYOND BOUNDARIES

10
Nursing Is Always Local

Tracy graduated with a doctoral degree in nursing from one of the world's leading universities. With her qualifications and publications in nursing's top journals in hand, she could have gotten an excellent academic position. Instead, she went to work as a pediatric nurse practitioner in a far-flung place where pediatric nursing was underdeveloped. She had the clinical skills and experience necessary to care for seriously ill young children in a resource-limited area, and after her doctoral study, she had the deep knowledge necessary to develop pediatric nursing in that hospital. And that is what she did. She did it, she said, because she felt compelled.

Before she left, I asked her why she did not apply for academic jobs locally. After all, I said, she had what it takes to make a difference here at home. As I was talking, she looked down at her hands. What I had said clearly bothered her. When I finished talking, she looked at me with frustration. "Mark," she said, "nursing is always local."

In bioethics, the tendency is to talk about the just distribution of health care resources. To talk about this, one needs boundaries, that is, countries—or within some countries, smaller regions such as states or provinces. Policymakers within these boundaries collect and redistribute resources, often based on local needs and sometimes based on political considerations. In this view, the locus of justice is the bounded state, as the contemporary philosopher Onora O'Neill says: the bounded state, a political entity, decides what is the just distribution of health care resources.

The obvious problem with this view is that health care problems do not know boundaries. We have seen this for centuries. In the fourteenth century, the plague moved from east to west and, in less than a decade, killed enough people that it took two hundred years for the world population to recover to its preplague levels. Today, with the warming climate, vector-borne diseases have traveled to places where before they were unseen, as I described in Chapter 8. It is easy to imagine communicable diseases crossing borders. But so do noncommunicable diseases.

The World Health Organization calls noncommunicable diseases—such as heart disease, cancer, diabetes, and chronic lung diseases—the major threat to the world's health. With modernization and urbanization, the world population has become more physically inactive. With the industrialization of agriculture, food production has become separated from its primary purpose of providing nutrients to the body. The tobacco industry, with its loss of major markets in high-income countries, has targeted advertising efforts in low-income countries. A 2016 study found that the number of tobacco advertisements was eighty-one times higher in low-income countries than in high-income countries. Consumption of alcohol, a known killer, is increasing worldwide, with the greatest increases of consumption—and the greatest increases of adverse effects on health—in low-income countries. And in high-income countries, opioid addiction rates soar, with overdose rates and deaths from overdose increasing year after year. Over seventy thousand people in the United States died from overdose in 2017 alone. The associated health care costs of the drug-use crisis for that year was almost $80 billion. As with communicable diseases, noncommunicable diseases travel without regard to borders.

In contrast with the notion of the bounded state as the locus of justice, a more useful concept of justice is based on the belief that we are one human community. Borders do not divide us. Mutual respect, as I discussed in the last chapter, is born out of our equal humanity. Equality, after all, is fairness, and as the twentieth-century philosopher John Rawls has written, fairness is justice. The answer to what is just when it comes to meeting the health challenges of the human community cannot depend on politically bounded societies. Rather, it has to come from bodies that stretch beyond borders, bodies that look at the health problems of the human community with respect to—that is, with respect for—humanity writ large. Nursing is one such body.

Nursing represents people from all over the world; it is as diverse as the world population. It is made up of individual nurses within groups of nurses that care for human communities all over the world. Ultimately, however, the profession of nursing is one global community of individual nurses who, in their collectivity, care for all people, regardless of boundaries.

This notion of the one human community is what the contemporary philosopher Anthony Kwame Appiah calls cosmopolitanism. Dating to the fourth century before the common era, the notion of cosmopolitanism means that, over and above our local loyalties, we are "citizens of the cosmos," that is, not just citizens of the globe but citizens of all that is. Nationalists have used the term "cosmopolitan" pejoratively. For example, in the mid-twentieth-century Soviet Union, "cosmopolitan" was used to label Jews as "antipatriotic." Near to the time of my writing this very sentence, an adviser to the US president accused a journalist of having a "cosmopolitan bias." By "cosmopolitan bias," the adviser meant that the journalist had extra-nationalist allegiances. I do not disagree that we are citizens of states, but to turn this adviser's use of "cosmopolitan bias" on its head, he was right: Our citizenship goes beyond the states whose passports we hold. We are citizens of the world. Just as the air we breathe knows no boundaries (we breathe the coal emissions from power plants far downwind); just as disease-carrying mosquitoes that have traveled from other, warmer climes bite us; just as we drink contaminated water from transboundary aquifers; and just as what one country does in the global economy is felt by other people on the far side of the globe, so too our obligations as nurses to the human community are unbounded. The cosmos is the locus of our nursing citizenship, and thus, our obligations stretch beyond the ties of formal, bounded citizenship. We are citizens of the one human community and of all that upon which the human community depends—the earth and the atmosphere above.

A central tenet of cosmopolitanism is that every human being has obligations to each other. In this book, I have argued that, as nurses, we have obligations to every human being, and these obligations are based in our unique function of promoting and restoring health through our care of the potentially sick, the sick, and the dying. I have chosen six obligations that, I think, are not enmeshed in particular societies. These obligations are not bounded by culture or by kith and kin. We have obligations to establish structures and to comport ourselves in ways that reflect human equality, to assist those who need it, to promote peace, to provide safety, to care for Earth, and to respect ourselves and each other. These obligations are universal to all nurses, and they are toward all people, including others who live outside the boundaries within which we find ourselves, for as nurses, we value all human life, even the life of strangers.

This was one aspect of what Tracy meant when she told me that all nursing is local: She was going to a place where she had not been before—a place where strangers lived. But their being strangers notwithstanding, she had obligations toward them. These strangers had a specific need that was matched by her knowledge and skills. She was going to fulfill her obligation to assist a particular community—a locality of strangers—that needed what she could give. She valued the lives of the people in that location. She was "going local," as it were, for long enough to fulfill her obligation. In fulfilling this obligation, she showed that she valued the particular human lives there. She took an interest in their particularities— their circumstances, their needs, and what she could do as a nurse to meet those needs. This was her obligation. We do have obligations to strangers, as Appiah says. This is what it means to be a cosmopolitan: to live out our obligations to strangers.

Such nursing exchanges, including exchanges of nursing students, are important because nurses from other localities can come to where we work and help us to improve our knowledge and skills, or learn from us. I have gone to countries in other parts of the world where the nursing care of people living with human immunodeficiency virus (HIV) was more developed than where I am from, and I have learned from them how to better provide HIV care. But these exchanges achieve far more than the transfer of knowledge and skills. In other countries, I have learned about the local nurses as humans—as people in their cultures, in their ways of life. These exchanges have helped me to understand the reasons that people—the nurses with whom I have worked and the people for whom they care—live the way they do. Understanding the reasons people in other localities live the way they do is part of respecting people who are not like us. These exchanges have also helped me to see, in the simplest but most profound ways, our commonalities: We eat different foods and drink different drinks, but we all eat and drink. We sleep on different surfaces and on different schedules and patterns, but we all sleep. We demonstrate our love in different ways, but we all love. And as we are dying, which we all do, we care about the same thing: having those we love around us. This is one of the great purposes of nursing exchanges: to create mutual respect, to create an awareness of our human equality. As I argued in Chapter 9, mutual respect leads us to treat each other fairly, and fair treatment is justice.

The other purpose of nursing exchanges is to see that we do not shoulder the entire burden of the world's problems. Appiah makes this point more strongly; he says that it is "our obligation not to carry the whole burden alone," for if we were to carry the burden alone, we would prevent others from doing their fair share.

Mutual respect and doing our fair share are two sides of the same coin. Mutual respect is treating each other fairly, but treating each other fairly means not doing for others what they are able—or need—to do for themselves. This, indeed, is the heart of Virginia Henderson's definition of nursing: we only do for others when they cannot do for themselves. This prevents us from a colonialist view of nursing, in which we lord our doing over others, preventing them from fulfilling their responsibilities to the human community. For instance, when one person does not do his or her fair share when he or she is able, he or she forces others to do it or others have to bear the consequences of his or her fair share not being done. Doing one's fair share also means that one cannot carry obligations that exceed one's capabilities. Rather, one must admit to one's limits and call upon others in the community to shoulder the burden.

Doing your fair share need not mean that you have to go to some far-flung location. You do your fair share where you are. This is another aspect of what it means for nursing to be local: whatever you construe your nursing obligations to be—the six I have argued for or an entirely different set—they must be achievable where you are. Appiah makes this point by quoting from George Eliot's 1876 novel *Daniel Derronda*. The main character in Eliot's novel, Daniel Derronda, is raised a Christian in England but finds out as an adult that he has Jewish ancestry. He responds to this discovery by saying that he has found "an added soul." Before this discovery, Derronda wandered "in the mazes of impartial sympathy." He was unmoved by the plight of an individual. People were just people. He himself was just a person. It was as if he had no one with whom he could identify. After discovering people with whom he could identify, he had an "added soul." And after finding this added soul, he chose "the noble partiality which is man's best strength, the closer fellowship that makes sympathy practical." That is, he understood that people have histories—and even plights, as the Jewish community has long had. He understood that he could not do good without knowledge of the needs of people close to him. This is the closer fellowship of which he speaks, the fellowship of the people where we are. We fulfill our nursing obligations where we are because that is where we can shoulder the burden with others—and do our fair share. It is where the closer fellowship makes shouldering the burden practical.

Appiah says that our obligations "must be consistent with our being . . . partial to those closest to us." The particularities of our ways of life—of our families, our friends, of "the many groups that call upon us through our identities"—demand partiality from us. My nursing obligations begin where I am, where I can fulfill them with those who give my life and the lives of those around me significance. Our obligations are to all humans, but also to particular human lives: my family, my community, and, more immediately, the patients who present to me in the place of care. We are also nurses of the specific countries (or states or provinces) that issue our licenses, and to them we owe our best nursing selves: we ought to take particular interest in fulfilling our obligations within the boundaries within which we are licensed.

However, as nurses, the worldwide nursing community gives us our identity, even though the state gives us our licenses. States have subjective conceptions of what is the just distribution of health care resources, for states have subjective conceptions of what is a good society. Any statist conception will inevitably favor one group of people over another. It will inevitably pit one's needs against another's. And it will end up in ambiguous statements about rights to this or that, rights that may not be compatible with other rights, and rights for which there may not be anyone to ensure enfranchisement. However, the worldwide profession of nursing, with an intellectually robust account of its obligations to the human community, does not speak with subjectivity, preference, or ambiguity. The nursing profession speaks as a collective of members of the human community, not as members of states.

If the worldwide profession of nursing reasoned about—and acted upon—basic obligations to support the well-being of its members, and if it did this in a way in which exchanges of knowledge, skills, and resources flowed freely to assist nurses to fulfill their obligations locally, in response to the local needs, then one can be a nurse in the closer fellowship that is one's local community while also being a nurse within the one human community. One can fulfill one's obligations locally and fulfill one's obligations to strangers by being a member of the profession. The profession allows us to fulfill our transboundary obligations. O'Neill suggests that the most effective agents of justice may be "different bodies and different institutions" than just the institutions of states. She lists nongovernmental organizations and religious groups as possibilities. But nursing, as the world's most populous health care profession situated everywhere around the world, is the body that can support the health of the world's population. Nursing is the body that, through fulfilling its obligations fairly, can be the agent of justice beyond boundaries.

Nursing is always local, as Tracy told me. Nursing is the patient in front of you, the community you live in, the state that licenses you, but also the transboundary environment that we use to heal the sick. And just as nursing is everywhere, so too can we justly support the well-being of the entire human community through nursing.

11

The Social Significance of Nursing

Books of this mood and genre usually end on a clarion note: the definition of what is good and what must be achieved. Authors often appear to assume that the work that needs to be done will follow, both in leadership and in policy if not in politics. If this work does not follow soon, they assume it will follow in due course, for having specified what the individual ought to do, the author's work is done; each reader must act from there. This optimism has sustained many an author in the belief that his or her clarion call will change the course of society.

I do not write with this type of optimism. Rather, I write with a nurse's optimism. It is a can-do optimism, an optimism that arises from nurses pulling together to do what needs to be done, even in what appear to be helpless circumstances. It is this optimism, a nurse's optimism, that gives up the idea of achieving perfect goodness, but rather finds goodness in the everyday work of caring.

I have seen this optimism in nurses everywhere. As I write these words, I am in India, having come to this country for the first time to speak at a conference. Inequality is more visible here, if not more prevalent, than in the United States. And tensions between different ethnoreligious groups can be felt. These tensions have erupted at various times, for example, as murders of others for being this or that religion and as acts of terror. Some of the people I have talked with feel voiceless and powerless to gain a voice. And yet, Indian nurses, just as nurses everywhere, care for people regardless of creed, ethnicity, caste, or, at the hospital where the conference was held, ability to pay. The nurses at this hospital practice radical equality. It is radical not just because it undoes what divides society, but also because, in the everyday act of nursing care, it augurs for peace and safety for all, as wars and violence can only arise when societies fracture along cultural, racial, ethnic, or class or caste lines—fractures that create inequality. These nurses have illustrated just how practical it is, in the closer fellowship, to work toward the common good through everyday nursing practice and how their practice calls others to fulfill their obligations to society. They illustrate that nurses can coalesce around a vision of the good society and work toward it—and this is radical: to find the goodness of equality in the everyday work of nursing.

However, there is more to do, these nurses told me, than care for the sick in hospitals. They told me about the programs they have initiated aimed at teaching people how to read, for literacy is necessary for health. Literacy also allows people to gain better employment, thereby reducing poverty. And, as many of the people the nurses are teaching to read are women, more literate women promotes gender equality. Just these two benefits alone—reduced poverty and improved gender equality—show that teaching people how to read is not just good for individual people's well-being; it is also good for the human community as a whole. These nurses' assistance of others, no matter how small scale, promotes the good society for all.

In the first chapter of this book, I envisioned a conference at which nurses from the earth's four corners would gather to address societal issues. I saw a glimpse of that possibility in these Indian nurses' efforts.

These sorts of efforts exist all around the world. Volunteer nurses staff health clinics for the homeless. Nurses from different countries join together to build capacity in each other's countries. Nurses call for a global ban on landmines as they care for victims. Nurses join with climatologists and environmental scientists to work for a healthier planet. These and other efforts are examples of how nurses, in small-scale efforts aimed at fulfilling their obligations, make the world a better place. To these nurses, a better world is not a thought exercise. It is everyday work they do.

I do not envision nursing as working toward a perfect world; rather, I envision it as working toward a better world. The idea that the perfect society consists entirely of people who look, think, and act alike pervades the age during which I write. It is an age that cannot tolerate difference. As I said in the preface, my time appears driven by the ideas of "Take my country back," of xenophobia, of exiling refugees from where we live, of believing that we, because we have placed a stake in the ground, have control over land that has been around for millennia and, hopefully, will be around long after we are gone. We do not control the air, the sea, the land, much less the inner workings of Earth and Earth's atmosphere. And in the age of global climate change, we cannot control where living organisms that transmit infectious diseases are able to travel. But we can control how we do and do not act. As nurses, we do not act as if we, by our care, usher in a perfect world—our perfect world, the world we want, *my* perfect world. No, I do not envision nursing working toward a perfect world.

Rather, nursing works toward a world in which the good of the action we can take in the moment is not sacrificed for the dream of perfection—perfection based in the ideas of exclusion and division, of personal gain and self-achievement. The good—in fact, I would say morality itself—is found in nurses' work in the imperfect world that is a reality. The good society is a dynamic process of doing here and now what needs to be done to make the world a *better* place.

This is the social significance of nursing: when in our everyday acts of nursing we fulfill obligations toward others—and toward Earth—we find a better world. A better world is, indeed, found in the doing.

Notes to Chapters

Foreword

"In May 2019, the World Health Assembly will declare 2020 as the 'Year of the Nurse and the Midwife'..."
World Health Organization 2019.

"As the cochair of the Nursing Now Global Campaign..."
Nursing Now 2019.

"In June 2019, at the International Council of Nurses (ICN) Congress in Singapore, the ICN will launch the Nightingale Challenge."
International Council of Nurses 2019b.

"...Agenda 2030, the United Nations' plan..."
United Nations 2015.

"...thirteen million hungry children living in the United States..."
US Department of Agriculture 2018.

"...nurses are the most trusted of all professions..."
M. Brennan 2018.

"Mary Wollstonecraft, with her 1792 *A Vindication of the Rights of Women*..."
Wollstonecraft 1988.

"Nightingale argued... that the profession of nursing was one way to do that."
Showalter 1981.

Chapter 1

"...one would expect them to be in the city having a good time after work."
J. M. Lazenby 2008.

"...Robert Bellah said..."
Bellah et al. 1991.

"..., the philosopher John Rawls, thought much the same ..." and "... must accept the principles by which these good political and social institutions operate ..."
Rawls 1999.

"The good society, according to ... John Kenneth Galbraith ..."
Galbraith 1996.

"Adam Smith, the eighteenth-century Scottish philosopher ..."
Smith 1878.

"... according to the Nobel economist and philosopher Amartya Sen ..."
Sen, 1985 2009a. Also see M. C. Nussbaum 2011.

"Florence Nightingale, pressed for reforms ..."
McDonald 2006.

"The contemporary social psychologist Dacher Keltner ..."
Keltner 2009.

"In nursing, knowledge about how to improve society meets application of that knowledge."
Goodrich 1932; Buhler-Wilkenson 2001.

"Lillian Wald, who lived as a nurse among poor immigrants in the tenements of New York City ..."
Wald 2015.

"In 1867, the American poet Emma Lazarus ..."
Lazarus 1944.

"... in Lazarus's 1883 poem, 'The New Colossus' ..."
Lazarus 1949.

Chapter 2

"... along with six million more Jews, a quarter-million people with disabilities, over two hundred thousand Roma, among many, many others ... "
The United States Holocaust Memorial Museum estimates that people who implemented the Nazi population policy during World War II killed nearly eighteen million people.
"... in 1948, the United Nations. . . . At the same time, the UN adopted the Universal Declaration of Human Rights."
United Nations General Assembly 1949.

"... Samantha Power, who has chronicled Lemkin's work ..."
Power 2002.

"... the American Nurses Association's and the International Council of
Nurses' codes of ethics ..."
American Nurses Association 2015; International Council of Nurses 2012.
The American Nurses Association's code of ethics states that respect for dignity is "the fundamental principle that underlies all nursing practice." The first
standard in the United Kingdom's Nursing and Midwifery Council's code of
professional standards involves upholding the dignity of people. The idea of
human dignity plays a foundational role in many other countries' nursing
associations and councils' codes of ethics, including Australia, New Zealand,
and South Africa.

"... Some philosophers, such as John Rawls ..."
Rawls 1999.

"... Simon Blackburn, does not even mention it ..."
Blackburn 2001.

"... Peter Singer, argues ..."
Singer 2015.

"The concept of dignity can be made to carry with it overtones of elitism ... or
be based in religious belief ..."
I am grateful to Leon Kass's 2017 work for these points.

"... the contemporary psychologist Steven Pinker ..."
Pinker 2008.

"The seventeenth-century philosopher John Locke understood the shame of
people ..."
Locke 1948.

"That equality is our common humanity."
Strauss 1950.

"This common humanity is the moral basis of our relationship with each
other."
Simmons 1992.

"... the eighteenth-century German philosopher Immanuel Kant ..."
Kant 1998, 1997a.

"Contemporary nurse scholars Susan Benedict and Linda Shields have chronicled..."
Benedict and Shields 2014.

"Nurses also participated in the crimes of apartheid."
Nonceba 2006.

"... non-Jewish nurses during the Holocaust..."
Yad Vashem, The World Holocaust Remembrance Center, 2018.
"... white nurses during apartheid..."
Jarrett-Kerr 2017.

"They say they did what they would have wanted others to do for them if their roles were reversed."
Mayer 2011.

Chapter 3

"... some economists think that eliminating cash..."
Rogoff 2014.

"Witness babies who begin to cry when they hear other babies cry."
Goleman 1989; Stern and Cassidy 2018.

"... if we help others in the way we would want anyone, including ourselves, to be helped."
Keltner 2016.

"In that use, the word carries with it a sense of debt."
See Shakespeare's use in *King Lear* (1623) Act II, Scene ii, line 314, and in *Hamlet* (1604) Act I, Scene ii, line 91.
"Cicero, the Roman philosopher..."
Cicero 2000, book 1, paragraph 22, pp. 9–10.

"We repay this debt by being honest, prudent, fair, temperate, and courageous."
The four virtues (prudence, fairness, termperance, and courage) are, to Cicero, the source of moral rightness. They have also been called the four cardinal virtues. See Cicero 2000, book 1, paragraph 15.

"... we repay our debt to virtue by developing in ourselves virtuous habits."
I have elsewhere discussed the moral habits we can cultivate in ourselves as a way of leading the good life as a nurse (M. Lazenby 2017).

"In this way, we cannot escape obligations."
M. Lazenby 2017, p. 76.

"Cicero thought that we have certain obligations that arise out of the roles we have in life . . ."
For the first two roles, see Cicero 2000, book 1, paragraph 107, p. 37.

"When we do, we owe a debt to ourselves . . . to do it well."
For the third and fourth roles, see Cicero 2000, book 1, paragraphs 115–116, pp. 38–39.

"People from many fields, not just nursing, have turned to science . . ."
Salovey 2016.

"Science may give us insight into the way the world works, but science cannot teach us how to live sustainably."
Ellis 2018b.

". . . these solutions have contributed to people's untimely deaths . . ."
This statement should be commonplace knowledge, at least since Rachel Carson's 1962 book *Silent Spring*.

". . . human uses of the scientific technologies of the industrial age."
US Environmental Protection Agency, 2017.

"But it also brings satisfaction to the doer."

On this notion of nursing as a calling, see M. Lazenby 2017, pp. 6–7. And see a wonderful 1997 article by Ritva Raatikainen.
"The twentieth-century nurse-theorist Virginia Henderson . . ."
Henderson 1969.

". . . when a person undertakes the work of nursing in the service of our common humanity . . ."
I have in mind here something akin to John Rawls's notion of justice as fairness arising out of some "Original Position," that is, the position from which we can discover the nature of justice and what it requires of us as individual persons and of the social institutions through which we will live together cooperatively (Rawls 1999).

". . . we have a social contract that arises from our discharging our debts to our shared humanity."
Our work as nurses on behalf of others, when viewed as a calling, is work that we need to do—it is work we are compelled to do. At the same time, the work that we do is work that needs to be done for the world to be a better place. So when we do the work of nursing, we do both what we need to do and work the world needs to have done. This is the very nature of a calling (M. Lazenby 2017,

pp. 6–7). When we do the work of nursing and the world becomes a better place through what we have done, we create in others a debt, an obligation. Their repayment of this obligation is that they do what they must to make the world a better place. This is the contract between nurse and patient, nurse and family, nurse and community, nurse and society. Nursing is by no means the only profession that has this social-contract aspect to it, but nursing must recognize this aspect of its profession, for it is in recognizing this aspect that nursing moves beyond the findings of its scientists to changing the world for the better.

"The choice to become a nurse necessarily involves taking a particular position in society, a position that carries with it a contract to care."
See Henning Mankell's (2016) discussion on p. 103 of his memoir *Quicksand: What It Means to Be a Human Being*, particularly this: "The choices a human being has to make also involve deciding where one stands in an unjust society: we are all political beings, whether we like it or not. We live in a fundamentally political society, where we have a sort of contract with everybody else who lives alongside us."

"Nightingale worked to improve . . ."
McDonald 2010.

"It is fashionable in nursing to rest the ethical behavior of nurses on promoting, advocating, and protecting the rights of patients, rights . . ."
See Provision 3 of the American Nurses Association's (ANA) code of ethics (American Nurses Association 2015). Notice also that the ANA has a Center for Ethics and Human Rights, the work of which is, in part, to increase nurses' "sensitivity to human rights" (American Nurses Association 2017).

"From this fashion has come campaigns for patients' bills of rights."
The American Hospital Association (AHA) first adopted the Patient's Bill of Rights in 1973, which the AHA has since come to call the Patient Care Partnership (American Hospital Association 2019).

". . . as the UN Universal Declaration of Human Rights proclaims."
See Articles 1 and 25 of the Universal Declaration of Human Rights, which was passed on December 10, 1948, by the United Nations in General Assembly Resolution 217 A (United Nations, General Assembly 1949).

". . . the contemporary British philosopher Onora O'Neill says."
O'Neill 2016, pp. 27–28.

"Simone Weil, a French philosopher . . ."
Weil 1952, p. 3.

"Obligations . . . are universal" and ". . . Weil's word, 'eternal.' "
Weil 1952, p. 4.

"Any nursing theory . . . begins with obligations."
O'Neill 2016, p. 38.

Chapter 4

Throughout this chapter I am indebted to the general lines of thought of Ronald Dworkin (2000).

"Armartya Sen says the good society gives individuals this freedom."
Sen 1999, 2009b.

"Nussbaum lists ten essential capacities . . ."
Nussbaum 2000.

"In Nussbaum's list is bodily integrity . . ."
Nussbaum 2000, 2011. The full list is:

1. Life—Able to live to the end of a normal-length human life, and to not have one's life reduced to not worth living.
2. Bodily Health—Able to have a good life that includes (but is not limited to) reproductive health, nourishment, and shelter.
3. Bodily Integrity—Able to change locations freely, in addition to having sovereignty over one's body, which includes being secure against assault (for example, sexual assault, child sexual abuse, domestic violence, and the opportunity for sexual satisfaction).
4. Senses, Imagination, and Thought—Able to use one's senses to imagine, think, and reason in a "truly human way"—informed by an adequate education. Furthermore, the ability to produce self-expressive works and engage in religious rituals without fear of political ramifications. The ability to have pleasurable experiences and avoid unnecessary pain. Finally, the ability to seek the meaning of life.
5. Emotions—Able to have attachments to things outside of ourselves; this includes being able to love others, grieve at the loss of loved ones, and be angry when it is justified.
6. Practical Reason—Able to form a conception of the good and critically reflect on it.
7. Affiliation—A. Able to live with and show concern for others, empathize with (and show compassion for) others, and the capability of justice

and friendship. Institutions help develop and protect forms of affiliation. B. Able to have self-respect and not be humiliated by others, that is, being treated with dignity and equal worth. This entails (at the very least) protections from being discriminated on the basis of race, sex, sexuality, religion, caste, ethnicity, and nationality. In work, this means entering relationships of mutual recognition.

8. Other Species—Able to have concern for and live with other animals, plants, and the environment at large.

9. Play—Able to laugh, play, and enjoy recreational activities.

10. Control over One's Environment—A. Political—Able to effectively participate in the political life, which includes having the right to free speech and association. B. Material—Able to own property, not just formally, but materially (that is, as a real opportunity). Furthermore, having the ability to seek employment on an equal basis as others, and the freedom from unwarranted search and seizure.

"... symmetrical in our possession of these capacities ..."
Rawls 1999, pp. 11, 130, 260. Also see Scarry 2001.

"... until our patients gain independence and can do those things for themselves."
Henderson 1964.

"According to the twentieth-century theologian Paul Tillich ..."
Tillich 1961, p. 100.

"The epidemiologists Richard Wilkinson and Kate Pickett ..."
Wilkinson and Pickett 2010. Also see Marmot 2015.

"Elizabeth Bradley and her colleagues at the Yale School of Public Health used state-level and national data ..."
Bradley 2016.

"... we should also think about investment in social services and public health."
Bradley et al. 2016, p. 767.

"Jessie Beard, a nurse writing in the *American Journal of Nursing* in 1917 ..."
Beard 2017.

"... and it is from her that our modern public health nursing and school nursing specialties arose."
Philips 1999.

"Wald too knew the truth..."
Wald 2015.

"... Mary Shaw, a medical sociologist, and Danny Dorling, a human geographer..."
Shaw and Dorling 2004.

"... and in their choice of where they live and work."
Shaw and Dorling 2004, p. 903.

"... of what physicians and surgeons earn."
According to the US Bureau of Statistics, in 2016, the annual mean salary for physicians and surgeons was $210,170, for nurse practitioners $104,610, and for registered nurses $72,180 (US Bureau of Statistics 2017).

"... according to the Nobel economists Robert Shiller and Joseph E. Stiglitz..."
Shiller 2016; Stiglitz 2012.

"... earns more than 184 times the income of 90 percent of everybody else."
Institute for Policy Studies n.d.

"... the top 1 percent of the wealthiest of society had more wealth than the rest of the world put together."
Dorling 2014. Also see Hardoon, Ayele, and Fuentes-Nieva 2016.

"... eight men had as much wealth as roughly 3.6 billion people..."
Hardoon 2017.

"... as sociologist Linsey McGoey..."
McGoey 2015. As companion volumes on the exploitive nature of the wealthiest of the wealthy, see Aschoff 2015, and Giridharadas 2018.

"... inequality... is widening worldwide..."
Hardoon 2017.

"... and in the history of the United States, it is at its greatest ever..."
Covert 2016.

"And as the top 1 percent hoard the world's wealth, the United States increasingly spends more on health care than on social services and public health..."
Bradley and Taylor 2013. Also see Rubin et al. 2016.

"Amartya Sen, in his 1983 book..."
Sen 1983.

Chapter 5

This is Virginia Henderson's definition of nursing (Henderson 1964).

This notion of treating others as we would like them to treat ourselves and other humans is Immanuel Kant's categorical imperative, which is that one should act as one would want all other people to act toward all other people. The best formulation of the categorical imperative is in section II of Kant's *Groundwork for the Metaphysics of Morals* (Kant 1997b). Simply put, a categorical imperative is that which we ought to do unconditionally. Of course, we have a choice whether or not to do that which we ought to do. However, if we do not do it, we are not moral people. I am claiming that, as nurses, assisting others is, for us, that which we ought to do.

This is Kant's notion of an "imperfect duty." It is imperfect because it admits of multiple means of achieving it. It would indeed be immoral to assist in a way that does more harm because you do not have the knowledge and skills necessary to provide the kind of assistance that is needed, but it would also be immoral that, if you did not have the knowledge and skills, you did not seek out those who did. That is, your assistance can come in the form of finding those who are able to provide the kind of assistance that the other needs. Even though the duty to assist is an imperfect duty, and hence, can be fulfilled in more than one way, it is still categorical: it is a duty you cannot shirk.

But I am tempted to think of the duty to assist as a perfect duty for nurses. Perfect duties, according to Kant, are those duties that one must always do. Nurses must assist others in those activities that restore or promote health or lead to a peaceful death. There is not one way to do this, of course, as there is only one way not to lie (a perfect duty). And in this sense, the duty to assist is imperfect. But because there is more than one way to fulfill the duty to assist does not get nurses out of assisting even if they do not have the knowledge and skills necessary. They still have the duties to assist in securing the people who have the requisite knowledge and skills.

". . . for as Nussbaum says, the moral life is based on a willingness to being exposed."
See Nussbaum 1968, part II.

"The family court judge overseeing her situation remarked . . ."
Royal Courts of Justice, the United Kingdom, 2017.

"... which has had more acquired immune deficiency syndrome (AIDS)-related deaths per capita than any other country in the Global North."
Engel 2006.

"... the Botswana Harvard AIDS Institute Partnership ..."
Harvard T. H. Chan School of Public Health 2019.

Chapter 6

"Exposed people were dying of cancer ..."
Simon, Bouville, and Land 2006.

"... the land remained radioactive, and thus, unsafe for life."
Vartabedian 2009.

"In 1973, the WHO held its first discussion on the threat nuclear war posed to health."
World Health Organization 1985, p. 121.

"... the Thirty-Fourth World Health Assembly passed resolution 34.38 ... "
World Health Organization 1985, p. 398.

"... the resolution, which affirmed that health and peace are inextricably connected, passed."
World Health Organization, 1985; see subcommittee B's seventh report.

"The photograph, taken by Mahmoud Raslan ..."
Raslan 2016.

"She casts her eyes downward."
Vonnow 2016.

"... for providing health care had been bombed out."
Boghani 2016.

"... the US Department of Veterans Affairs registered almost one million disability claims related to these wars."
Watson Institute: International & Public Affairs, Brown University, 2019.

"... had been forcibly displaced worldwide because of violence or war."
United Nations High Commissioner for Refugees 2015.

"... according to the contemporary essayist Elaine Scarry ..."
Scarry 2014, Chapter 3, pp. 157–188.

"Scarry writes that Locke 'was . . . and precision.' "
Scarry 2014, p. 158.

"Scarry puts it this way: . . . 'body.' "
Scarry 2014, p. 158.

". . . what he called the 'miserable condition of war.' "
Hobbes 1994, Chapter 17, p. 223.

" 'The social contract,' Scarry says, 'is a contract for peace.' "
Scarry 2014, p. 158.

". . . we need for 'commodious living' and the hope of having the means to obtain these things."
Hobbes 1994, p. 188.

"But life becomes large when we live peaceably with each other."
See Annette Baier's classic and very important 1987 article, "Commodious Living."

". . . what Scarry calls 'the equality of aliveness.' "
Scarry 2014, p. 164.

". . . everywhere 'to seek peace, and follow it,' to use Hobbes's phrase."
Hobbes 1994, Chapter 14, p. 190.

". . . the American Nurses Association's code of ethics."
American Nurses Association 2015.

Chapter 7

". . . Wislawa Szymborska illustrates in his 1998 poem 'Conversation with a Stone' . . ."
Szymborska 2001.

"As a civil society, we recognize that there are members of society who . . . need our protection more."
The source of this idea is a great New Zealand nurse, Irihapeti Ramsden (1990).

". . . those who most hold social and political power."
Bailey 2017.

"It is, as Martha Nussbaum says, 'the basic social emotion' . . ."
Nussbaum 1996, p. 35.

"We see ourselves as people to whom such things might happen in the future."
Nussbaum 1996.

"Compassion is also thinking about what humans ought to have by virtue of being human."
Nussbaum 1996, p. 33.

"As clergyman and antiwar activist William Sloane Coffin Jr. said . . ."
Coffin 1973.

"Compassion, in nursing, means holding everything together."
M. Lazenby 2017, p. 57.

Chapter 8

". . . scientists have named this geologic age the Anthropocene."
International Commission on Stratigraphy 2015.

". . . Paul Crutzen, first proposed the concept of the 'Anthropocene' . . ."
Steffen et al. 2011, p. 843.

"It is only with the Industrial Revolution that the human community exited this relationship, and the Anthropocene began in earnest."
Steffen et al. 2011.

"Steffen, Grinevald, Crutzen, and McNeill detail the dramatic increase in such atmospheric-imprinting human activity in a now-legendary 2011 article." "This accelerated activity's effect on the global environment is clearly discernable, Steffen, Grinevald, Crutzen, and McNeill say." And "They warn: If the human activities that drive the Anthropocene . . ."
Steffen et al. 2011, pp. 848 and 862.

". . . the United Nations' Intergovernmental Panel on Climate Change has just released a scientific report that describes the consequences of the already-warming climate . . ."
Intergovernmental Panel on Climate Change (IPCC) 2018.

". . . the US Global Change Research Program issued a startling report on these health effects."
US Global Change Research Program 2016.

". . . they disproportionately face the loss of means of living, and loss of life it-self, from extreme weather events related to the warming climate."
Mal et al. 2018.

"They will lose their means of food production, their livelihoods, and their lives more than the rich."
World Bank and Potsdam Institute for Climate Impact Research and Climate Analytics 2017.

". . . ancestral villages have been lost to the rising sea, traditional ways of life have been forever altered, and poverty has increased from the loss of fishing livelihoods."
Bronen 2013.

". . . Alaska Natives have been among the poorest people in the United States."
US Census Bureau 2018.

"Their fate will one day be the fate of all, rich and poor alike."
World Bank 2010.

"Florence Nightingale . . . [i]n her 1860 *Notes on Nursing* . . ."
Nightingale (1860) 2011.

". . . water clean . . ." and "air pure . . ."
Nightingale (1860) 2011, see pp. 8, 27, 30, 102, 107, 127, 129, 13r-136.

". . . according to a US government study . . . is filled with high levels of toxic chemicals."
Agency for Toxic Substances and Disease Registry, Division of Toxicology and Human Health Sciences, Environmental Toxicology Branch, 2018.

"We are in the process of changing Earth's inherent nature."
A. Brennan 1984.

"The profession's leading association, the International Council of Nurses (ICN), has done this."
International Council of Nurses 2018.

"Environmental ethics (that is, our obligation to Earth) is to work 'together across all our diverse and unequal social worlds,' as . . . Ellis says."
Ellis 2018a, 2018b.

". . . we can call the health care industry to lead by example."
Jameton 2009.

". . . Emmanuel Vaughan-Lee interviews these men about their experience."
Vaughn-Lee 2018.

Chapter 9

"Gordon Kamara was an ambulance nurse in Monrovia, Liberia . . ."
Solomon 2014.

" . . . the primacy of the good of caring for the potentially sick, the sick, and the dying."
M. Lazenby 2017.

"Self-respect, according to the philosopher John Rawls, is the confidence . . ."
and "At first, this seems a tautology, an empty truth."
Stark 2012, pp. 238–261.

" . . . and when his or her performance is thus, he or she is an expert."
Benner 1984.

Chapter 10

"In this view, the locus of justice is the bounded state, the philosopher Onora O'Neill says . . ."
O'Neill 2016.

"The World Health Organization calls noncommunicable diseases . . . the major threat to the world's health."
Chan 2017.

" . . . eighty-one times higher in low-income countries than in high-income countries."
Savell et al. 2015.

"Consumption of alcohol, a known killer . . ."
Wood et al. 2018.

" . . . and the greatest increases of adverse effects on health—in low-income countries."
World Health Organization 2018.

" . . . with overdose rates and deaths from overdose increasing year after year" and "Over seventy thousand people in the United States died from overdose in 2017 alone."
CDC/NCHS, 2018.

"The associated health care costs of the drug-use crisis for that year was almost $80 billion."
Florence et al. 2016.

". . . what the contemporary philosopher Anthony Kwame Appiah calls cosmopolitanism."
Appiah 2006, p. 174.

"For example, in the mid-twentieth-century Soviet Union, 'cosmopolitan' was used to label Jews as 'antipatriotic.' "
Figes 2007.

". . . an adviser to the US president accused a journalist of having a 'cosmopolitan bias.' "
Ben-Ghiat 2017.

". . . just as we drink contaminated water from transboundary aquifers . . . "
Rivera 2015.

"We do have obligations to strangers, as Appiah says" and "Appiah makes this point more strongly; he says that it is 'our obligation not to carry the whole burden alone.' "
Appiah 2006, pp. 153 and 164.

"This . . . is the heart of Virginia Henderson's definition of nursing."
Henderson 1964.

"George Eliot's 1876 novel *Daniel Derronda* . . ."
Eliot 1995, pp. 661–662.

"Appiah says that our obligations 'must be consistent with our being . . . partial to those closest to us' . . of 'the many groups that call upon us through our identities' . . ."
Appiah 2006, p. 165.

"O'Neill suggests that the most effective agents of justice may be 'different bodies and different institutions' . . ."
O'Neill 2016, p. 223.

Bibliography

AARP Foundation and the Robert Wood Johnson Foundation. n.d. *Campaign for Action*. Accessed November 11, 2018. https://campaignforaction.org/.

Agency for Toxic Substances and Disease Registry, Division of Toxicology and Human Health Sciences, Environmental Toxicology Branch. 2018. *Toxicological Profile for Perfluoroaklyls*. Washington, DC: US Department of Health and Human Services.

American Hospital Association. 2019. *The Patient Care Partnership*. Accessed January 20, 2019. https://www.nursingworld.org/practice-policy/nursing-excellence/ethics/.

American Nurses Association. 2015. *Code of Ethics for Nurses with Interpretive Statements*. Silver Spring, MD: American Nurses Association.

———. 2017. *Ethics and Human Rights*. Accessed January 20, 2018. https://www.nursingworld.org/practice-policy/nursing-excellence/ethics/.

Appiah, Kwame Anthony. 2006. *Cosmopolitanism: Ethics in a World of Strangers*. New York: W. W. Norton & Company.

Arias, M. E., E. Lee, F. Farinosi, F. F. Pereira, and P. R. Moorcroft. 2018. "Decoupling the Effects of Deforestation and Climate Variability in the Tapajós River Basin in the Brazilian Amazon." *Hydrological Processes* 32: 1648–1663.

Aschoff, Nicole. 2015. *The New Prophets of Capital*. London: Verso Gooks.

Baier, Annette C. 1987. "Commodious Living." *Synthese* 72 (2): 157–185.

Bailey, Zinzi, Nancy Krieger, Madina Agénor, Jasmine Graves, and Natalia Linos. 2017. "Structural Racism and Health Inequities in the USA: Evidence and Interventions." *The Lancet* 389 (10077): 1453–1463.

Beard, Jessie L. 2017. "The Correlation Between Nursing and Social Work." *American Journal of Nursing* 18 (1): 21–24.

Bellah, Robert, Richard Madsen, William M. Sullivan, Ann Swindon, and Steven M. Tipton. 1991. *The Good Society*. New York: Knobf Press.

Benedict, Susan, and Linda Shields. 2014. *Nurses and Midwives in Nazi Germany: The Euthanasia Programs*. New York: Routledge, Taylor & Francis Group.

Ben-Ghiat, Ruth. 2017. *CNN Opinion: Loaded Word of the Week: Cosmopolitan*. August 4. Accessed January 15, 2019. https://www.cnn.com/2017/08/04/opinions/cosmopolitan-bias-immigration-opinion-ben-ghiat/index.html.

Benner, Patricia. 1984. *From Novice to Expert: Excellence and Power in Clinical Nursing Practice.* Menlo Park, CA: Addison-Wesley.

Bennett, D., D. C. Bellinger, L. S. Birnbaum, A. Bradman, A. Chen, D. A. Cory-Slechta, S. M. Engel, et al. 2016. "Project TENDR: Targeting Environmental Neuro-Developmental Risks: The TENDR Consensus Statement." *Environmental Health Perspectives* 124 (7): A118–A122.

Berlin, Isaiah. 2001. *The Power of Ideas.* London: Pimlico.

Blackburn, Simon. 2001. *Being Good: An Introduction to Ethics.* Oxford: Oxford University Press.

Boghani, Priyanka. 2016. *Frontline: Syria at War.* February 11. Accessed January 20, 2019. https://www.pbs.org/wgbh/frontline/article/a-staggering-new-death-toll-for-syrias-war-470000/.

Bradley, E., M. Canavan, E. Rogan, K. Talbert-Slagle, C. Ndumele, L. Taylor, and L. Curry. 2016. "Variation in Health Outcomes: The Role of Spending on Social Services, Public Health, and Health Care, 2000–09." *Health Affairs* 35 (5): 760–768.

Bradley, Elizabeth H., and Lauren A. Taylor. 2013. *The American Health Care Paradox: Why Spending More Is Getting Us Less.* New York: PublicAffairs.

Brennan, Andrew. 1984. "The Moral Standing of Natural Objects." *Environmental Ethics* 6 (1): 35–56.

Brennan, Megan. 2018. "Nurses Again Outpace Other Professions for Honesty, Ethics." December 20. Accessed February 2, 2019. https://news.gallup.com/poll/245597/nurses-again-outpace-professions-honesty-ethics.aspx.

Bronen, Robin. 2013. *Climate-Induced Displacement of Alaska Native Communities.* Washington, DC: Brookings Institution.

Buhler-Wilkenson, Karen. 2001. *No Place Like Home: A History of Nursing and Home Care in the United States.* Baltimore: Johns Hopkins University Press.

Carson, Rachel. 1962. *Silent Spring.* New York: Houghton Mifflin.

Cattani, D., V. L. de Liz Oliveira Cavalli, C. E. Heinz Rieg, J. T. Domingues, T. Dal-Cim, C. I. Tasca, F. R. M. B. Silva, and A. Zamoner. 2014. "Mechanisms Underlying the Neurotoxicity Induced by Glyphosate-Based Herbicide in Immature Rat Hippocampus: Involvement of Glutamate Excitotoxicity." *Toxicology* 320: 34–45.

CDC/NCHS. 2018. *National Vital Statistics System, Mortality.* December 18. Accessed December 2018. https://wonder.cdc.gov/.

Centers for Disease Control and Prevention. 2018. *Illnesses on the Rise from Mosquito, Tick and Flea Bites.* May 1. Accessed September 29, 2018. https://www.cdc.gov/vitalsigns/vector-borne/index.html.

Chan, Margaret. 2017. "Non-Communicable Diseases: The Slow-Motion Disaster." In *Ten Years in Public Health 2007–2017: A Report Dr. Margaret*

Chan, Director-General, World Health Organization, 91–106. Geneva: World Health Organization.

Cicero. 2000. *On Obligations*. Translated with an introduction and notes by P. G. Walsh. Oxford: Oxford University Press.

Coffin, William Sloan. 1973. "Prayer for the 50th Anniversary of Yale School of Nursing." Chaplain's Office, Yale University.

Covert, Bryce. 2016. *Income Inequality Is at the Highest Level in American History*. ThinkProgress. July 1. Accessed January 2019. https://thinkprogress.org/income-inequality-is-at-the-highest-level-in-american-history-d2c263980be6.

Crichton, Michael. 1990. *Jurassic Park*. New York: Alfred A. Knopf.

Dabla-Norris, Era, Kapla Kochlar, Nuin Suphaphiphat, Frantisek Ricka, and Evridiki Tsounta. 2015. *Causes and Consequences of Income Inequality: A Global Perspective*. International Monetary Fund. June 5. Accessed February 2019. https://www.imf.org/en/Publications/Issues/2016/12/31/Causes-and-Consequences-of-Income-Inequality-A-Global-Perspective-42986.

Daegan, Michael. 2018. *This Radical Land: A Natural History of American Dissent*. Chicago: University of Chicago Press.

DellaValle, Curt. 2015. *Rethinking Carcinogenesis: New View of Cancer Development Focuses on Subtle, Combined Effects*. Washington, DC: Environmental Working Group.

Diamond, Cora. 1991. "Experimenting on Animals: A Problem in Ethics." In *The Realistic Spirit: Wittgenstein, Philosophy, and the Mind*, 355–66 Cambridge, MA: MIT Press.

Doocy, S., A. Daniels, S. Murray, and T. D. Kirsch. 2013. "The Human Impact of Floods: A Historical Review of Events of 1980–2009 and Systematic Literature Review." *PLOS Current Disasters*. April 16. doi:10.1371/currents.dis.f4deb457904936b07c09daa98ee8171a.

Dorling, Danny. 2014. *Inequality and the 1%*. New York: Verso.

Dow Chemical. 2012. *Agent Orange*. August 23. Accessed September 2, 2018. https://www.dow.com/en-us/about-dow/issues-and-challenges/agent-orange.

Dworkin, Ronald. 2000. *Sovereign Virtue: The Theory and Practice of Equality*. Cambridge, MA: Harvard University Press.

Eliot, George. 1995. *Daniel Derronda*. London: Penguin.

Ellis, Erle C. 2018a. *The Anthropocene: A Short Introduction*. Oxford: Oxford University Press.

———. 2018b. "What Kind of Planet Do We Want?" *New York Times*, August 12, SR1.

Engel, Jonathan. 2006. *The Epidemic: The Global History of AIDS*. New York: Harper Collins.

Figes, Orlando. 2007. *The Whisperers: Private Life in Stalin's Russia*. New York: Metropolitan Books.

Florence, C. S., C. Zhou, F. Luo, and L. Xu. 2016. "The Economic Burden of Prescription Opioid Overdose, Abuse, and Dependence in the United States, 2013." *Medical Care* 54 (10): 901–906.

Galbraith, John. 1996. *The Good Society: The Humane Agenda*. Boston: Houghton Mifflin Co.

Giridharadas, Anand. 2018. *Winners Take All: The Elite Charade of Changing the World*. New York: Knopf.

Goleman, Daniel. 1989. "Researchers Trace Empathy's Roots to Infancy." *New York Times*, March 28, C1.

Goodrich, Annie Warburton. 1932. *The Social and Ethical Significance of Nursing*. New York: The Macmillan Company.

Guha-Sapir, Debarati, Philippe Hoyois, Pasacline Wallemacq, and Regina Below. 2016. *Annual Disaster Statistical Review 2016: The Numbers and Trends*. Brussels: Centre for Research on the Epidemiology of Disasters.

Hamra, G. B., F. Laken, A. J. Cohen, O. Raaschou-Nielsen, M. Brauer, and D. Loomis. 2015. "Lung Cancer and Exposure to Nitrogen Dioxide and Traffic: A Systematic Review and Meta-Analysis." *Environmental Health Perspectives* 123: 1107.

Hardoon, Deborah. 2017. *An Economy for the 99%*. January. Accessed June 17, 2017. https://www.oxfam.org/sites/www.oxfam.org/files/file_attachments/bp-economy-for-99-percent-160117-summ-en.pdf.

Hardoon, Deborah, Sophia Ayele, and Ricardo Fuentes-Nieva. 2016. *An Economy for the 1%: How Privilege and Power in the Economy Drive Extreme Inequality and How This Can Be Stopped*. January 18. Accessed January 20, 2019. https://oxf.am/2FKbYYL.

Harvard T. H. Chan School of Public Health. 2019. *Botswana Harvard Partnership*. Accessed January 20, 2019. https://aids.harvard.edu/research/bhp/.

Henderson, V. 1964. "The Nature of Nursing." *American Journal of Nursing* 64 (4): 62–68.

Henderson, Virginia. 1969. "Excellence in Nursing." *American Journal of Nursing* 69 (10): 2133–2137.

Hillebrand, H., T. Brey, J. Gutt, W. Hagen, K. Metfies, B. Meyer, and A. Lewandowska. 2018. "Climate Change: Warming Impacts on Marine Biodiversity." In *Handbook on Marine Environment Protection: Science, Impacts and Sustainable Management*, edited by Markus Salomon and Till Markus, 355–73. New York: Springer International Publishing.

Hobbes, Thomas. 1994. *Leviathan: With Selected Variants from the Latin Edition of 1668*. Indianapolis, IN: Hackett Publishing Company.

Hystad, P., P. J. Villenueve, M. S. Goldberg, D. L. Crouse, and K. Johnson. 2015. "Exposure to Traffic-Related Air Pollution and the Risk of Developing Breast Cancer Among Women in Eight Canadian Provinces: A Case-Control Study." *Environmental International* 74: 240–248.

Institute for Policy Studies. n.d. *Income Inequality.* Accessed June 17, 2017. http://inequality.org/income-inequality/.

Intergovernmental Panel on Climate Change (IPCC). 2018. *Global Warming of 1.5 °C: An IPCC Special Report on the Impacts of Global Warming of 1.5 °C Above Pre-Industrial Levels and Related Global Greenhouse Gas Emission Pathways, in the Context of Strengthening the Global Response to the Threat of Climate Change.* Nairobi, Kenya: United Nations Environmental Programme.

International Agency for Research on Cancer, World Health Organization. 2012. *Cancer Fact Sheets.* Accessed September 1, 2018. http://gco.iarc.fr/today/fact-sheets-cancers?cancer=29&type=0&sex=0.

International Commission on Stratigraphy. 2015. *International Chronostratigraphic Chart v2015/01.* Accessed September 2, 2018. http://www.stratigraphy.org/ICSchart/ChronostratChart2015-01.pdf.

International Council of Nurses. 2012. *The ICN Code of Ethics for Nurses.* Geneva: International Council of Nurses.

———. 2018. *Nurses, Climate Change and Health.* Position Statement. Geneva, Switzerland: International Council of Nurses.

———. 2019a. *Voice to Lead.* Accessed January 20, 2019. https://www.icnvoicetolead.com/.

———. 2019b. *One Year Since the Launch of the Nursing Now Campaign.* Accessed April 15, 2019. https://www.icn.ch/news/one-year-launch-nursing-now-campaign.

Jameton, Andrew. 2009. "Medicine's Role in Mitigating the Effects of Climate Change." *Virtual Mentor* 11 (6): 465–469.

Jarrett-Kerr, Martin. 2017. *Apartheid in Nursing: A Challenge: An African Nurse.* Accessed September 2018. https://www.sahistory.org.za/archive/apartheid-in-nursing-a-challenge-an-african-nurse.

Johnson & Johnson Services. 2018. *Nurses Change Lives.* May 30. Accessed November 11, 2018. https://nursing.jnj.com/home.

Kant, Immanuel. 1997a. *Critique of Practical Reason.* Edited by Mark Gregor. Cambridge: Cambridge University Press.

———. 1997b. *Groundwork for the Metaphysics of Morals.* Translated and edited by Mary Gregor, with an introduction by Christine M. Korsgaard. Cambridge: Cambridge University Press.

———. 1998. *Groundwork of the Metaphysics of Morals.* Edited by Mary Gregor. Cambridge: Cambridge University Press.

Kass, Leon. 2017. *Leading a Worthy Life: Finding Meaning in Modern Times*. New York: Encounter Books.

Keltner, Dacher. 2009. *Born to Be Good: The Science of a Meaningful Life*. New York: W. W. Norton & Company.

———. 2016. *The Power Paradox: How We Gain and Lose Influence*. New York: Penguin Press.

Keynes, John Maynard. 1936. *The General Theory of Employment, Interest, and Money*. London: Palgrave Macmillan.

Lazarus, Emma. 1944. *Emma Lazarus: Selections from Her Poetry and Prose*. Edited by Jewish Peoples Fraternal Order Morris U. Schappes and International Workers Order. New York: Cooperative Book League, Jewish American Section.

———. 1949. *The New Colossus*. Washington, DC: Library of Congress; Philip and Fanny Duschnes.

Lazenby, James Mark. 2008. "The Face of Health Care." *American Journal of Nursing* 108: 72JJ–72KK.

Lazenby, Mark. 2017. *Caring Matters Most: The Ethical Significance of Nursing*. New York: Oxford University Press.

Leibniz, Gottfried. 2015. *Leibniz, Gottfried Wilhelm: Sämtliche Schriften und Briefe*. Berlin: Degruyter.

Locke, John. 1948. *The Second Treatise of Civil Government*. Oxford: Basil Blackwell.

Kahneman, Daniel. 2011. *Thinking, Fast and Slow*. New York: Farrar, Strauss and Giroux.

Mal, S., R. B. Bingh, C. Huggel, and A. Grover. 2018. "Introducing Linkages Between Climate Change, Extreme Events, and Disaster Risk Reduction." In *Climate Change, Extreme Events and Disaster Risk Reduction*, edited by Suraj Mal, R. B. Singh, and Christian Huggel, 1–14. New York: Springer International Publishing.

Mankell, Henning. 2016. *Quicksand: What It Means to Be a Human Being*. Translated by Laurie Thompson. New York: Vintage Books.

Marmot, Michael. 2015. *The Health Gap: The Challenge of an Unequal World*. New York: Bloomsbury Press.

Mayer, Jack H. 2011. *Life in a Jar: The Irena Sendler Project*. Middlebury, VT: Long Trail Press.

McDonald, Lynn. 2006. *Florence Nightingale: As a Social Reformer*. January 1. Accessed September 1, 2018. https://www.historytoday.com/lynn-mcdonald/florence-nightingale-social-reformer.

———. 2010. *Florence Nightingale: At First Hand*. Waterloo, Ontario, Canada: Wilfrid Laurier University Press.

McGoey, Linsey. 2015. *No Such Thing as a Free Gift: The Gates Foundation and the Price of Philanthropy.* London: Verso Books.

Melillo, Jerry M., Terese (T. C.) Richmond, and Gary W. Yohe, eds. 2014. *Climate Change Impacts in the United States: The Third National Climate Assessment.* Washington, DC: US Global Change Research Program.

Nightingale, Florence. (1860) 2011. *Notes on Nursing: What It Is, and What It Is Not.* Cambridge: Cambridge University Press.

Nonceba, Lubanga. 2006. "Human Rights Violation in Health: The Legacy of Apartheid in Nursing." Paper presented at the *134th Annual Meeting of the American Public Health Association*, Boston.

Nursing Now. 2019. *Nursing Now.* Accessed April 15, 2019. https://www.nursingnow.org/.

Nussbaum, Martha. 1986. *The Fragility of Goodness: Luck and Ethics in Greek Tragedy and Philosophy.* Cambridge: Cambridge University Press.

———. 1996. "Compassion: The Basic Social Emotion." *Social Philosophy and Policy* 13 (1): 27–58.

———. 2000. *Women and Human Development: The Capabilities Approach.* New Delhi: Kali for Women.

———. 2011. *Creating Capabilities: The Human Development Approach.* Cambridge, MA: Belknap Press of Harvard University Press.

O'Neill, Onora. 2016. *Justice Across Boundaries: Whose Obligations?* Cambridge: Cambridge University Press.

Philips, Deborah. 1999. "Healthy Heroines: Sue Barton, Lillian Wald, Lavinia Lloyd Dock and the Henry Street Settlement." *Journal of American Studies* 33 (3): 65–82.

Pinker, Steven. 2008. *The Stupidity of Dignity.* May 28. Accessed September 2018. https://newrepublic.com/article/64674/the-stupidity-dignity.

Power, Samantha. 2002. *"A Problem from Hell": American and the Age of Genocide.* New York: Basic Books.

Raatikainen, Ritva. 1997. "Nursing Care as a Calling." *Journal of Advanced Nursing* 25: 1111–1115.

Ramsden, Irihapeti. 1990. "Cultural Safety." *New Zealand Nursing Journal* 83 (11): 18–19.

Ramsfield, T. D., B. J. Bentz, M. Faccoli, H. Jactel, and E. G. Brockerhoff. 2016. "Forest Health in a Changing World: Effects of Globalization and Climate Change on Forest Insect and Pathogen Impacts." *Forestry: An International Journal of Forest Research* 89: 245–252.

Raslan, Mahmoud. 2016. *Five-Year-Old Syrian Omran Daqneesh.* Aleppo, Syria: Aleppo Media Center.

Rawls, John. 1999. *A Theory of Justice.* Cambridge, MA: Belknap Press of Harvard University Press.

Redeker, K. R., L. L. Cai, A. J. Dumbrell, A. Paul, J. Bardill, J. Chong, and T. Helgason. 2018. "Noninvasive Analysis of the Soil Microbiome: Biomonitoring Strategies Using the Volatilome, Community Analysis, and Environmental Data." *Advances in Ecological Research* 59:93–132.

Rivera, A. 2015. "Transboundary Aquifers Along the Canada–USA Border: Science, Policy and Social Issues." *Journal of Hydrology: Regional Studies* 4, Part B: 623–643.

Rogoff, Kenneth. 2014. *Costs and Benefits to Phasing Out Paper Currency.* May 16. Accessed January 20, 2018. http://scholar.harvard.edu/files/rogoff/files/c13431.pdf.

Roundtable on Environmental Health Sciences, Research, and Medicine, Board on Population Health and Public Health Practice, and Institute of Medicine. 2014. *Identifying and Reducing Environmental Health Risks of Chemicals in Our Society: Workshop Summary.* Washington, DC: National Academies Press.

Roy, Nicole M., Bruno Carneiro, and Jeremy Ochs. 2016. "Glyphosate Induces Neurotoxicity in Zebrafish." *Environmental Toxicology and Pharmacology* 42: 45–54.

Royal Courts of Justice, the United Kingdom. 2017. Neutral Citation Number [2017] EWHC 2036 (Fam) (High Court of Justice Family Division). August 3. https://www.scribd.com/document/355434666/Neutral-Citation-Number-2017-EWHC-2036-Fam

Rubin, Jennifer, Jirka Taylor, Joachim Krapels, Alex Sutherland, Melissa Felician, Jodi Lui, Lois Davis, and Charlene Rohr. 2016. *Are Better Health Outcomes Related to Social Expenditure? A Cross-National Empirical Analysis of Social Expenditure and Population Health Measures.* Santa Monica, CA: RAND Corporation. http://www.rand.org/content/dam/rand/pubs/research_reports/RR1200/RR1252/RAND_RR1252.pdf.

Salovey, Peter. 2016. "University Priorities and Academic Investments." Email communication to the Yale University Faculty. November 21. New Haven, CT: Yale University.

Savell, Emily, Anna B. Gilmore, Michelle Sims, Prem K. Mony, Teo Koon, Khalid Yusoff, Scott A. Lear, et al. 2015. "The Environmental Profile of a Community's Health: A Cross-Sectional Study on Tobacco Marketing in 16 Countries." *Bulletin of the World Health Organization* 93:851–861.

Scarry, Elaine. 2001. *On Beauty and Being Just.* Princeton, NJ: Princeton University Press.

————. 2014. *Thermonuclear Monarchy: Choosing Between Democracy and Doom*. New York: W. W. Norton.

Sen, Amartya. 1983. *Poverty and Famines: An Essay on Entitlement and Deprivation*. Oxford: Oxford University Press.

————. 1985. *Commodities and Capabilities*. Amsterdam: North-Holland.

————. 1999. *Commodities and Capabilities*. New York: Oxford University Press.

————. 2009a. *The Idea of Justice*. Cambridge, MA: Belknap Press of Harvard University Press.

————. 2009b. *The Standard of Living: Tanner Lectures in Human Values*. Cambridge: Cambridge University Press.

Shaw, Mary, and Danny Dorling. 2004. "Who Cares in England and Wales? The Positive Care Law: Cross-Sectional Study." *British Journal of General Practice* 54 (509): 899–903.

Shiller, Robert. 2016. "Inequality Today, Catastrophe Tomorrow." *New York Times*, August 28. Edition BU4.

Showalter, Elaine. 1981. "Florence Nightingale's Feminist Complaint: Women, Religion and 'Suggestions for Thought.'" *Signs* 6 (3): 395–412.

Simmons, John A. 1992. *The Lockean Theory of Rights*. Princeton, NJ: Princeton University Press.

Simon, Steven, André Bouville, and Charles E. Land. 2006. "Fallout from Nuclear Weapons Tests and Cancer Risks: Exposures 50 Years Ago Still Have Health Implications Today That Will Continue into the Future." *American Scientist* 94 (1): 48–57.

Singer, Peter. 2015. "Is the Sanctity of Life Ethic Terminally Ill?" In *Bioethics: An Anthology*, edited by Helga Kuhse, Udo Schüklenk, and Peter Singer, 321–30. Hoboken, NJ: Wiley-Blackwell.

Smith, Adam. 1878. *An Inquiry into the Nature and Causes of the Wealth of Nations*. New York: R. Worthington.

Solomon, Ben C. 2014. "Life and Death Through the Eyes of an Ebola Nurse." *New York Times*, October 16. https://www.nytimes.com/times-insider/2014/10/16/life-and-death-through-the-eyes-of-an-ebola-crew/.

Spielberg, Steven, dir. 1993. *Jurassic Park*. Universal City, CA: Universal Pictures.

Stark, Cynthia. 2012. "Rawlsian Self-Respect." In *Oxford Studies in Normative Ethics*, edited by Mark Timmons, 2:238–261. New York: Oxford University Press.

Steffen, Will, Jacques Grinevald, Paul Crutzen, and John McNeill. 2011. "The Anthropocene: Conceptual and Historical Perspectives." *Philosophical Transactions of the Royal Society* 369: 842–867.

Stern, Jessica A., and Jude Cassidy. 2018. "Empathy from Infancy to Adolescence: An Attachment Perspective on the Development of Individual Differences." *Developmental Review* 47: 1–22.

Stiglitz, Joseph E. 2012. *The Price of Inequality: How Today's Divided Society Endangers our Future.* New York: W. W. Norton & Company.

Strauss, Leo. 1950. *Natural Right and History.* Chicago: University of Chicago Press.

Szymborska, Wislawa. 2001. "Conversation with a Stone." *Kenyon Review* 23 (2): 90–93.

Temkin, Alex, and the Environmental Working Group. 2018. *Breakfast with a Dose of Roundup?* August 15. Accessed September 2, 2018. https://www.ewg.org/childrenshealth/glyphosateincereal/#.W4vJUthKjBK.

Tillich, Paul. 1961. "The Meaning of Health." *Perspectives in Biology and Medicine* 5 (2): 92–100.

United Nations. 2015. *Transforming Our World: The 2030 Agenda for Sustainable Development.* September 25. Accessed April 15, 2019. https://sustainabledevelopment.un.org/post2015/transformingourworld.

United Nations, General Assembly. 1949. *The University Declaration of Human Rights.* New York: King Typographic Service Corporation.

United Nations High Commissioner for Refugees. 2015. *Global Trends Forced Displacement 2015.* Accessed January 20, 2019. https://www.unhcr.org/576408cd7.pdf.

US Bureau of Statistics. 2017. *May 2016 National Occupational Employment and Wage Estimates.* March 31. Accessed June 17, 2017. https://www.bls.gov/oes/current/oes_stru.htm.

US Census Bureau. 2018. *Facts for Features: American Indian and Alaska Native Heritage Month: November 2015.* August 3. Accessed October 6, 2018. https://www.census.gov/newsroom/facts-for-features/2015/cb15-ff22.html.

US Department of Agriculture. 2018. *Food Security Status of U.S. Households in 2017.* September 5. Accessed February 7, 2019. https://www.ers.usda.gov/topics/food-nutrition-assistance/food-security-in-the-us/key-statistics-graphics.aspx.

US Environmental Protection Agency. 2017. *Global Greenhouse Gas Emissions Data.* April 17. Accessed September 2, 2018. https://www.epa.gov/ghgemissions/global-greenhouse-gas-emissions-data.

US Environmental Protection Agency. 2017. *Causes of Climate Change.* Accessed February 12, 2017. https://19january2017snapshot.epa.gov/climate-change-science/causes-climate-change.html.

US Global Change Research Program. 2016. *The Impacts of Climate Change on Human Health in the United States: A Scientific Assessment.* Washington, DC: US Global Change Research Program.

Vartabedian, Ralph. 2009. "Nevada's Hidden Ocean of Radiation." *Los Angeles Times,* November 13. http://articles.latimes.com/2009/nov/13/nation/na-radiation-nevada13/2.

Vaughn-Lee, Emmanuel. 2018. "A First Glimpse of Our Magnificent Earth, Seen from the Moon." *New York Times,* October 2. https://www.nytimes.com/2018/10/02/opinion/earthrise-moon-space-nasa.html?action=click&module=Opinion&pgtype=Homepage.

von Ruette, J., P. Lehmann, and D. Or. 2018. "Quantifying Deforestation Effects on Rainfall Induced Shallow Landslides and Debris Flows Pathways." *EGU General Assembly Conference Abstracts 20th Edition.* 11465.

Vonnow, Brittany. 2016. "STRIFE THROUGH A LENS: Photographer Who Took THAT Picture of Bombed Aleppo Boy Reveals the Harrowing Story Behind the Iconic Image." *The Sun,* August 19. https://www.thesun.co.uk/news/1639805/photographer-who-took-that-picture-of-bombed-aleppo-boy-reveals-the-harrowing-story-behind-the-iconic-image/.

Wald, Lillian. 2015. *The House on Henry Street.* New York: Henry Holt and Company.

Watson Institute: International & Public Affairs, Brown University. 2019. *Costs of War: Executive Summary.* Accessed January 20, 2019. https://watson.brown.edu/costsofwar/.

Weil, Simone. 1952. *The Need for Roots: Prelude to a Declaration of Duties Towards Mankind.* Preface by T. S. Eliot. London: Routledge.

Wilkinson, Richard, and Kate Pickett. 2010. *The Spirit Level: Why Greater Equality Makes Societies Stronger.* New York: Bloomsbury Press.

Wollstonecraft, Mary. 1988. *A Vindication of the Rights of Women.* New York: Norton.

Wood, Angela M., Stephen Kaptoge, Adam S. Butterworth, Peter Willeit, Samantha Warnakula, Thomas Bolton, Ellie Paige, et al. 2018. "Risk Thresholds for Alcohol Consumption: Combined Analysis of Individual-Participant Data for 599 912 Current Drinkers in 83 Prospective Studies." *The Lancet* 391 (10129): 14–20.

World Bank. 2010. *The Impact of Climate Change on Cities.* Washington, DC: World Bank.

World Bank and Potsdam Institute for Climate Impact Research and Climate Analytics. 2017. *Turn Down the Heat: Climate Extremes, Regional Impacts and the Case for Resilience.* Washington, DC: World Bank.

World Health Organization. 1985. *Handbook of Resolutions and Decisions, 1973–1984.* Vol. 2. Geneva: World Health Organization.

———. 2018. *Global Status Report on Alcohol and Health 2018.* Geneva: World Health Organization.

———. 2019. *Executive Board Designates 2020 as the "Year of the Nurse and Midwife."* January 19. Accessed April 15, 2019. https://www.who.int/hrh/news/2019/2020year-of-nurses/en/.

World Health Organization, International Agency for Research on Cancer. 2018. *IARC Monographs on the Evaluation of Carcinogenic Risks to Humans.* July 30. Accessed September 2, 2018. https://monographs.iarc.fr/agents-classified-by-the-iarc/.

Wu, S., S. Powers, W. Zhu, and Y. A. Hannun. 2015. "Substantial Contribution of Extrinsic Risk Factors to Cancer Development." *Nature* 529: 43.

Yad Vashem, The World Holocaust Remembrance Center. 2018. *Bronislava Krištopavičienė.* Accessed September 1, 2018. http://www.yadvashem.org/yv/en/exhibitions/righteous-women/kristopaviciene.asp.

Yi, S.-W., and H. Ohrr. 2014. "Agent Orange Exposure and Cancer Incidence in Korean Vietnam Veterans: A Prospective Cohort Study." *Cancer* 120 (23): 3699–3706.

Discussion Questions

Chapter 1: Nursing and the Good Society

1. I have identified Sen's capabilities approach—the approach that says that the good society is bound up in people having the freedom to be and to do that of which they are capable—as necessary for the good society. What do you think is necessary for a good society?
2. How does your work as a nurse bring about this necessary aspect?
3. Describe the context in which you work, and, in your description, identify forces that pull you toward caring for others and forces that pull toward care-lessness, that is, the absence of caring.
4. What image serves for you as an image of good nursing, that is, an image of a nurse who makes the world a better place?

Chapter 2: Nursing and Our Common Humanity

1. When you have felt disrespected by another person, what about being disrespected hurt the most? How would you relate this thing that hurt the most to that which you share with others?
2. How might you respond to someone, especially a patient, who disrespected you?
3. How would your response help that person to see his or her own disrespect toward him- or herself?
4. How does your nursing practice embody the notions that dignity equals and respect recognizes our common humanity?

Chapter 3: Nursing and Obligation

1. How would you define the concept of obligation? Compare and contrast your definition with the chapter's understanding of the concept.
2. Do you agree with the argument that nurses have obligations toward all of humanity? Give your reasons for your agreement or disagreement.

3. What do you think is the relationship between human rights and humans' obligations toward each other?
4. How does your nursing practice fit into this relationship?

Chapter 4: Equality

1. How would you define equality?
2. How does your definition relate to your work as a nurse?
3. Based on your nursing experience, if you could influence governmental policies around social and public health spending, what programs would you want the government to increase funding for?
4. Which entity, governments or philanthropic organizations, is best suited to promote social equality? Give reasons for your answer.
5. If you won a very large lottery jackpot (as in the hundreds of millions), would you rather have fewer taxes on it to give more of it to philanthropic organizations, or would you rather governments choose how to spend that tax amount?

Chapter 5: Assistance

1. Did you know, when you became a nurse, how being a nurse would require you to assist others?
2. Recall a story of a patient whose care you did not want to assist in. Why did you not want to assist this patient? What does this not wanting to assist say about your estimation of the patient's humanity?
3. Think of a time in which you needed assistance and received it (or did not receive it). How did this make you feel about you as a person?
4. How has assisting a patient exposed you to the uncertainties of the world? And how have you felt about yourself when you have felt exposed to these uncertainties?

Chapter 6: Peace

1. Relate the promotion of peace in the context of war to the promotion of peace in the conflicts you experience in caring for your patients. How does promoting peace in internecine conflicts, or in conflicts between health care providers, promote health?

2. Describe an experience you have had in caring for a patient during which you knew that you were making the possibilities of the patient's life larger (or more commodious). How does this experience give you an insight into the profession's possibility of reducing violence and war?

3. The word "radical" means to affect the fundamental nature of something. How has your nursing practice radically affected others' lives for the better?

Chapter 7: Safety

1. Have you experienced the safety of a nurse caring for you? How can you extrapolate from this experience to the thought of the profession providing safety for the most vulnerable of society?

2. If you have ever experienced a structural inequality, how did this experience feel? What did you want others to do to ameliorate this feeling?

3. Would ameliorating this feeling have addressed the inequality? If so, how? If not, why not?

Chapter 8: Earth

1. Describe how you use Earth and its atmosphere in caring for patients, along the lines of Nightingale's theory.

2. Describe a patient for whom you have cared whose reason for being in your care was related, directly or indirectly, to the environment. How does this patient's story motivate you to care for the environment?

3. Read the International Council of Nurses' Position Statement, "Nurses, Climate Change and Health." What can you do at your institution and in your everyday role to promote Earth's health?

Chapter 9: Respect

1. What is your plan for your life as a nurse? Are you confident that this plan is worthy of your carrying out?

2. Describe a time when you felt confident in what you were doing as a nurse. How did this confidence affect other areas of your practice?

3. Remember an experience when you did not feel mutual respect between a colleague and you. Why did this experience feel the way it did to you?

Did both of you share your reasons for why you acted the way you did? How could you have repaired (or did you repair) this sense of a lack of mutual respect with this colleague?

Chapter 10: Nursing Is Always Local

1. Describe caring for a patient who was from a different part of the world and who spoke a different language. How did you relate with this patient? In what way did this experience bring another part of the world to you?
2. In what ways are nurses first citizens of the world and then citizens of their countries?
3. If you could go on a nursing exchange, even if you have practiced for many years, where would you want to go? Why there? What would you hope to get from this exchange?

Chapter 11: The Social Significance of Nursing

1. For what reasons are you optimistic that nursing can effect social change?
2. What, to you, makes up the good society?
3. How do you think your practice as a nurse works toward the good society?

APPENDIX

International Council of Nurses Position Statement

Nurses, Climate Change and Health

Climate change presents the single largest threat to global development with the potential to undermine the past 50 years of public health gains.[1] Nurses can make a powerful contribution to both mitigate climate change and to support people and communities around the world to adapt to its impacts. Leadership from nurses to take immediate action to build climate resilient health systems is necessary. This includes, but is not limited to, developing models of care to reduce unnecessary travel, developing climate-informed health programmes for emerging infectious and communicable diseases; engaging in sustainable practices in the health sector, building the response capacity of the health workforce; engaging in health and climate research, and participating in intersectoral policy and governance responses.[1] The healthcare sector makes both positive and negative contributions to climate change. The nursing profession has a duty to contribute to climate change adaptation (reducing vulnerability to the harmful effects) and mitigation (reducing or preventing greenhouse gas (GHG) emissions) as it is committed to protecting health and wellbeing and to promoting social justice.

Climate change refers to a change in the state of the climate which is attributed directly or indirectly to human activity that alter the composition of the global atmosphere and which is in addition to natural climate variability observed over a comparable period.[2] Climate change is unequivocal: the atmosphere and oceans have warmed, the quantity of snow and ice has diminished and the sea levels have risen.[3]

Climate change is a direct result of the rise in global concentrations of greenhouse gases (GHGs) in the atmosphere. These human-induced GHG emissions arise out of use of natural resources, particularly in the energy, transport, industry, agriculture, forestry and land use sectors.[3] To reduce climate change and protect health and wellbeing, a reduction in GHG emission is required and only through international cooperation and commitment to mitigation and adaptation strategies will this be accomplished. [4] The Paris

Agreement (2016) aims to achieve this through strengthening the global response to climate change and at the time of writing 179 Parties have ratified.[5] The effects of climate change have profound implications for human health and wellbeing. The adverse effects will arise from an impact on our most fundamental determinants of health: food, water, air and a safe environment that enables protection from extreme weather events. Health is already affected and the impacts are expected to increase as climate variability and change continue. The World Health Organisation (WHO) predicts that between 2030 and 2050, climate change is expected to cause approximately 250,000 additional deaths per year from malnutrition, malaria, diarrhoea and heat stress.[4] According to the Lancet Commission "the delayed response to climate change over the past 25 years has jeopardised human life and livelihoods" and has created potentially irreversible human symptoms.[1]

The relationship between health and climate change is complex. The mechanisms through which health is affected are both direct: heat-related incidents, extreme temperatures and extreme weather events (floods, drought, storms) and indirect: water quality, air pollution, land use change, and ecological changes. These mechanisms interact with certain social dynamics to produce negative health outcomes. Social dynamics include age, gender, health status, socioeconomic status, social capital, public health infrastructure and mobility and conflict status. The resulting impact on health and wellbeing includes loss of livelihoods, mental illness, increased food- and water-borne infections; increased vector- borne diseases; respiratory and cardiovascular diseases, and undernutrition.[1,3]

All regions and populations will be affected but those who will be displaced by the effects of climate change and people in low- and middle-income countries, are disproportionately affected.[1,3,4,6] This vulnerability will be further challenged by lowered resilience, less access to resources and decreased capacity to adapt and respond to the threats of climate change.[7] The susceptibility of countries to the adverse effects of climate change depends on factors such as topography, population density, economic and infrastructure development, food availability, income level and distributions, local environmental conditions, and the quality and availability of primary healthcare. At the population level, groups that are already considered disadvantaged and vulnerable—young children, older people, women (70% of the 1.3 billion people living in poverty, people with existing health problems or disabilities, poor and marginalised communities and indigenous populations—are most at risk for adverse health and wellbeing outcomes associated with climate change.[1] Indigenous populations are not only affected by the impacts of climate change but also by some mitigation strategies. Furthermore, their ability to adapt is compromised by legal, political, technical and financial contexts.[8]

Improving core public health infrastructure services (clean water, sanitation), ensuring essential health care (vaccination and child health services) and improving disaster preparedness and response capacities will have the most effective impact on reducing risks in the near term.[5] Climate informed strategies also have the potential to directly reduce risks to health, enhance community resilience, alleviate poverty, and address global inequities.[3]

Increased demand for well-educated and trained nurses is likely to occur as the incidence and prevalence of non-communicable diseases (NCDs) is rising across the globe. When coupled with the trend towards ageing populations, climate change is likely to further increase the demand for nurses capable of caring for increasing populations of people with progressing and debilitating NCDs. The need for nurses to deliver integrated models of care—across promotion, prevention and management and control of lifestyle factors to prevent or delay progressing morbidity from NCDs—will be significant.

Disasters as a result of climate change are increasing in frequency and intensity. As such, nursing's existing collaborations and partnerships with humanitarian organisations will become even more important as the challenges and adverse health impact from disasters, coupled with displacement, will be complex and long-term.

As the global voice of nursing, ICN:

- Urges countries, who have not yet done so, to ratify the Paris Agreement without further delay.
- Strongly believes that nurses have a shared responsibility to sustain and protect the natural environment from depletion, pollution, degradation and destruction.
- Recognises that building climate change resilience must include efforts to improve and sustain the social and environmental determinants of health through sustainable development.[3,11]
- Recognises the opportunity to take advantage of the massive potential to implement mitigation and adaptation policies that also have co-benefits to health.[1]
- Calls on governments to scale-up financing for climate resilient health systems including developing models for healthcare workers to engage in sustainable practices. Donor countries should ensure that low- and middle-income countries are supported to strengthen their health systems and to reduce the environmental impact of healthcare.[3]
- Encourages governments to reduce the risks they are expected to face from climate change by making choices in how they advance technology and industry and make investments in infrastructure and public policies that have less environmental impact. This includes:
  • Well-designed urban transport systems to reduce use of motorized vehicles and promote active transport to reduce urban air pollution and support physical activity and mental health.[1,3]

- Housing with efficient insulation and protection from extreme weather events to cut energy consumption, reduce exposure to cold and heat, reduce infectious and vector-borne diseases, and in some countries, reduce the need for burning of biomass fuels and associated indoor air pollution.[1,3]
- Policies and support for individual choices that moderate consumption of animal products to reduce the associated significant GHG emissions and non- communicable disease burden 6
- Calls on governments to invest in climate change and public health research, monitoring, and surveillance to improve understanding of the health co-benefits of climate mitigation and the health implications of adaptation measures at the community and national levels.[1,3]

ICN encourages national nurses' associations (NNAs), in collaboration with their respective government, to:

- Work to enable nursing leadership and nurses to support healthcare organisations to contribute to climate change mitigation through implementation of environmental policies and sustainable practices.
- Engage in national and multisectoral measures to mitigate the impact of climate change on the population with a focus on vulnerable groups and those more exposed to disease and injury.
- Be involved in developing national action plans and policies for mitigation, adaptation, and resilience strategies as well as contribute to environmental health and justice policy-making.
- Raise awareness of the health implications of climate change and how to assess and address climate change risks to health by developing policy documents on the subject.
- Embed the concept of sustainability in nursing practice as well as climate change- related knowledge into nursing curricula and in post-registration continuing education.
- Collaborate with other health professional organisations, intergovernmental organisations, environmental and health organisations and other civil society groups when developing health-adaptation policies and programmes.
- Engage with media to promote public awareness of the harmful effects of climate change on health and to promote mitigation strategies.
- Support the introduction of incentives for nurses to incorporate environmentally responsible health practices into their interventions.
- Strengthen existing and create new partnerships with humanitarian organisations and other NNAs to increase collaborative action.

ICN calls on individual nurses in their role as clinicians, educators, researchers, policy influencers, or executives, to:

- Advocate for policies that promote the reduction of healthcare waste and ensure correct waste management.
- Actively engage in environmental health committees and policy-making that focus on the safety and protection of health workers and the management and regulation of the healthcare environment.
- Empower individuals, families and communities to make healthy lifestyle choices and change own practices (i.e. active transportation, use green energy, dietary changes) to decrease the contribution to GHGs.
- Engage with other sectors to support strategies that lower GHGs such as urban redesign, enhanced public transportation and modifying indoor technologies (i.e. cookstoves) to reduce emissions.
- Work with communities to build resilience to the impacts of climate change in a way that is driven by the local context and needs and that goes beyond reactivity but seeks to address underlying vulnerabilities. Strategies include vulnerability assessments to develop resilience plans, incorporating uncertainty in resilience planning, including poor and socially excluded groups into decision making, scaling successful adaption interventions, and monitoring and evaluation.[12]

Adopted in 2008
Revised in 2018

References

1. Watts N, Neil Adger W, Agnolucci P, et al. Health and climate change: policy responses to protect Public health. Lancet [Internet]. 2015 [cited 2018 Jul 17]; 386:1861–914. Available from: https://doi.org/10.1016/S0140-6736(15)60854-6.
2. United Nations. United Nations Framework Convention on Climate Change (UNFCCC) [Internet]. New York: United Nations; 1992 May 9 [cited 2018 Jul 17]. Available from: https://unfccc.int/files/essential_background/background_publications_htmlpdf/application/pdf/conveng.pdf
3. Intergovernmental Panel on Climate Change (IPCC). Climate change 2014: Synthesis report. Contribution of Working Groups, I, II, III to the Fifth Assessment Report of the Intergovernmental Panel on Climate Change [Core writing team, Pachauri RK, Meyer LA (eds.)]. Geneva: IPCC; 2014 [cited 2018 Jul 17]. Available from: http://www.ipcc.ch/report/ar5/syr/
4. World Health Organisation (WHO). Climate Change and health: Fact Sheet [Internet]. Geneva: World Health Organisation; 2017 [cited 2018

Jul 17]. Available from: http://www.euro.who.int/__data/assets/pdf_file/ 0007/347983/13-Fact-sheet-SDG-Climate-change-FINAL-25-10-2017. pdf?ua=1.

5. United Nations. Paris Agreement. [Internet]. New York: United Nations; 2015 Dec 12 [cited 2018 Jul 17]. Available from:https://unfccc.int/sites/de-fault/files/english_paris_agreement.pdf

6. World Health Organisation (WHO). Climate and health country profiles—2015: A global overview 2015. [Internet]. Geneva: World Health Organisation; 2015 [cited 2018 Jul 17]. Available from: http://apps.who. int/iris/bitstream/10665/208855/1/WHO_FWC_PHE_EPE_15.01_eng. pdf?ua=1

7. Food and Agriculture Organization of the United Nations (FAO). FAO's work on climate change: United Nations Climate Change Conference 2017. [Internet]. Rome: FAO; 2017 [cited 2018 Jul 17]. Available from: http://www.fao.org/3/a-i8037e.pdf

8. Oviedo G, Fincke A. Indigenous peoples and climate change. [Internet]. Brussels: European Parliament; 2009 May 13 [cited 2018 Jul 17]. Available from: https://cmsdata.iucn.org/downloads/european_parliament_study_on_indigenous_peoples_and_cli mate_change.pdf

9. Chung JW, Meltzer DO. Estimate of the carbon footprint of the US health care sector. JAMA [Internet]. 2009 Nov 11 [cited 2018 Jul 17]; 302(18):1970–1972. Available from: https://doi.org/10.1001/ jama.2009.1610

10. Sustainable Development Unit. Carbon footprint update for NHS in England: 2015. [Internet]. Cambridge: Sustainable Development Unit; 2016 Jan [cited 2018 Jul 17]. Available from: https://www.sduhealth.org. uk/policy-strategy/reporting/nhs-carbon-footprint.aspx.

11. World Health Organization (WHO). Strengthening health resilience to climate change: Technical briefing for the World Health Organization conference on health and climate.[Internet] Geneva: World Health Organization; 2015 [cited 2018 Jul 17]. Available from: http://www.who. int/phe/climate/conference_briefing_1_healthresilience_27aug.pdf

12. Chaudhury M. Strategies for reducing vulnerability and building resilience to environmental and natural disasters in developing countries. [Internet]. DC: World Resources Institute; 2017 [cited 2018 Jul 17]. Available from: https://www.un.org/development/desa/dspd/wp-content/uploads/sites/22/2017/04/Moushumi-Chaudhury-Strategies-to-Reduce-Vulnerability-Paper_WRI_Final.pdf. Copyright © 2018 by ICN—International Council of Nurses, 3, place Jean-Marteau, 1201 Geneva, Switzerland. Reprinted by permission.

Index

For the benefit of digital users, indexed terms that span two pages (e.g., 52–53) may, on occasion, appear on only one of those pages.